WOMEN'S HEALTH IN POST-SOVIET RUSSIA

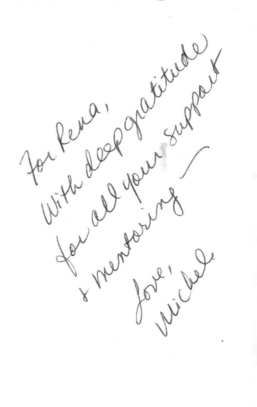

For Rena,
With deep gratitude
for all your support
& mentoring —
love,
Michele

NEW ANTHROPOLOGIES OF EUROPE

EDITORS

Daphne Berdahl, Matti Bunzl, and Michael Herzfeld

Women's Health in Post-Soviet Russia

The Politics of Intervention

MICHELE RIVKIN-FISH

Indiana University Press

Bloomington and Indianapolis

This book is a publication of

Indiana University Press
601 North Morton Street
Bloomington, IN 47404-3797 USA

http://iupress.indiana.edu

Telephone orders   800-842-6796
Fax orders   812-855-7931
Orders by e-mail   iuporder@indiana.edu

© 2005 by Michele Rivkin-Fish

The paper used in this publication meets the minimum requirements
of American National Standard for Information Sciences—
Permanence of Paper for Printed Library Materials, ANSI Z39.48-1984.

Manufactured in the United States of America

Library of Congress Cataloging-in-Publication Data

Rivkin-Fish, Michele R., date
  Women's health in post-Soviet Russia : the politics of intervention /
Michele Rivkin-Fish.
       p.   cm. — (New anthropologies of Europe)
  Includes bibliographical references and index.
  ISBN 0-253-34580-4 (cloth : alk. paper) — ISBN 0-253-21767-9
(pbk. : alk. paper)
     1. Women—Health and hygiene—Russia (Federation) 2. Maternal
health services—Russia (Federation) 3. Women's health services—
Russia (Federation) 4. Medical policy—Russia (Federation) I. Title.
II. Series.
  RA564.85.R56 2005
  362.1'082'0947—dc22   2005003117

1 2 3 4 5 10 09 08 07 06 05

For Ziggy, Itai, Sophie, and Natasha

In your book, you definitely should include the words of B.G. (Boris Grebenschikov):

Everything I do is an attempt to live like a human being, in conditions that are inhumane.

Vse to, shto ia delaiu, eto popytka zhit' po-chelovecheski, v nechelovecheskikh usloviiakh.

—my friend Karina, in a letter dated December, 2003

CONTENTS

ACKNOWLEDGMENTS

The generosity and support of numerous people made this book possible. First, I thank the women and health care providers in St. Petersburg, Russia, who willingly shared their stories and lives with me. I have tried my best to do justice to their experiences and perspectives, with the hope that the resulting accounts may help create more effective collaborations between people from around the globe who care about improving women's opportunities and well-being.

Several institutions made it possible for this study to be conducted, and I acknowledge them here with gratitude: research in 1993, 1994–95, and 1996 was sponsored by the Andrew C. Mellon Foundation, Princeton University, the Council on Regional Studies at Princeton, the Peter B. Lewis Fund of the Center of International Studies at Princeton, and a Princeton University Graduate Fellowship. Dissertation writing in 1996–97 was supported by a generous fellowship from the Mellon Foundation, Princeton University. Additional research in St. Petersburg in 2000 was funded by the International Research and Exchanges Board (IREX) and a University of Kentucky Summer Faculty Research Fellowship, for which I am grateful. I also acknowledge the assistance of the MacArthur Foundation, which provided additional research support during my collaboration with Andrej Popov and the Transnational Family Research Institute, Moscow, in 1995. Fieldwork in St. Petersburg in 1994–95 was conducted under the auspices of the Healthy Cities Project in Copenhagen, and I express my sincere gratitude to Dr. Agis Tsorous of WHO for his support.

My trajectory in becoming an anthropologist has led me to many special people who have enriched my life in immeasurable ways. Kevin Lourie gave me my first opportunity to conduct fieldwork with Russian speakers, igniting an interest and commitment that spanned much longer than either he or I could have imagined. A Maguire Fellowship from Vassar College enabled further research with Soviet immigrants in Israel just as the Soviet Union collapsed. The experiences I had and the friends I met in Jerusalem in 1990–91 convinced me that studying Russia would be an enormously rewarding, life-altering challenge. Later, faculty from Princeton University, including Rena Lederman, Vincanne Adams, Emily Martin, and Laura Engelstein, provided invaluable academic support. Loy Carrington, Lauren Leve, Nicole Monnier, Lawrence Rosen, Natasha Reed, and especially Carol Zanca offered friendship and practical assistance at several crucial junctions along the way. I am also grateful for having participated in the Rutgers University Center for Russian, Central, and East European Studies year-long seminar, Locations of Gender: Central and Eastern Europe. Discussions with other fellows in this seminar helped me refine several parts of this study.

While living in Russia, I received the support of the St. Petersburg Public Health Committee, including its International Department and WHO-Project Office. I particularly thank Elena Tkachenko for her hospitality and friendship. I am grateful to Lenya Shtutin and the Shtutin family for their enormous help in St. Petersburg with computers and apartments, and for all their generous practical and emotional support. My typist, Marina, did an excellent job transcribing thousands of hours of taped lectures, interviews, and conversations and was always a delight to work with. Natasha and Sergei Ivanov, Anya Popova, Sergei Zakharov and Galina Rakhmanova, and Sasha and Valera Tolkachev welcomed me into their homes to live during various periods of fieldwork and gave me the calming sense of being settled that can be so evasive during extended research trips. Irina Pchenichnikova was a pleasure to work with on the paid maternity care interviews, and I greatly appreciate all her efforts.

My colleagues at the University of Kentucky have assisted me in developing parts of the argument, and I gratefully thank Mary Anglin, Deb Crooks, Lisa Cliggett, Peter Little, Karen Petrone, Ellen Rosenman, Jean-Marie Rouhier-Willoughby, Nancy Schoenberg, and Gretchen Starr-LeBeau. Colleagues and friends in other universities and research settings also offered crucial assistance in helping me conceptualize my questions and formulate the analysis here. David Abramson, Julie Brown, Henry David, Elizabeth Dunn, Nanatte Funk, Bruce Grant, Igor Semenovich Kon, Maggie Paxson, Andrej Popov, Galina Rakhmanova, Kate Schecter, Judy Twigg, and Sergei Zakharov helped in key moments of the writing process. I thank Risto Alapuro, Johann Bachman, Katia Beloousova, Elizabeth Dunn, Susan Gal, Linda Gordon, Marcia Inhorn, Gail Kligman, Alena Ledeneva, Morgan Liu, Markku Lonkilla, Heather Paxson, Adriana Petryna, Natasha Reed, Katherine Verdery, Andrei Vinogradov, Catherine Wanner, and Alexei Yurchak for pushing me to think in critical ways and for provocative, helpful discussions.

The University of Michigan's Center for Russian and East European Studies provided a delightful and stimulating atmosphere for writing the bulk of this manuscript. I thank Barbara Anderson for inviting me and the U of M's CREES, International Institute, and School of Public Health

(Department of Health Behavior and Health Education) for hosting me. I am particularly grateful to Katherine Verdery, Deborah Field, Elena Gapova, and Alaina Lemon for welcoming me in Ann Arbor and providing valuable suggestions on earlier drafts of the text, and to Marcia Inhorn, Morgan Liu, Alan Pollard, and Elisha Renne for their wonderful support while I was writing.

Several friends read and commented on early drafts of the work and greatly helped me refine my analysis: Melissa Caldwell, Nanette Funk, Sergei Zakharov, Deborah Field, Larissa Remennick, and Otniel E. Dror all provided important suggestions and assistance. Special appreciation goes to Julie Hemment, who generously read and commented on numerous sections of this text, discussing them in painstaking detail with me on repeated occasions. I also thank Daphne Berdahl, Matti Bunzl, and Michael Herzfeld for their support of this project, and my editor at Indiana University Press, Rebecca Tolen, for all her help. I deeply appreciate the insightful and constructive comments of Alaina Lemon and Adriana Petryna.

Finally, the support I received from family and friends was essential for my ability to persevere throughout the ten years this project has taken. I thank Debbey Altman-Diamant, Bonnie Chernin, Elena Domatova, Michal Frenkel, Beth Goldstein, Julie Hemment, Natasha Ivanova, and Jodi Sandfort for always being there, and my parents, Betty Noble and Jerry Miller, and my brother and sister-in-law, Jason and Lita Miller, for always believing in me and lending all their support. My son, Itai, added a wonderful new dimension to my fieldwork in 2000, and my daughter Sophie made everyday life delightful during the revisions and final editing stages. My husband, Ziggy, supported this project in infinite intellectual, practical, and emotional ways from beginning to end, giving unlimited support on matters ranging from his skills with computers to his knowledge of Bourdieu and being constantly willing to read my drafts and listen to my concerns. There simply aren't words to express my thanks and love to him.

Portions of this book have appeared elsewhere in different forms, and I acknowledge the publishers of those articles here with gratitude for granting permission for me to include these materials here.

Parts of Chapter 1 appeared in "Health Development Meets the End of State Socialism: Visions of Democratization, Women's Health, and Social Well-Being for Contemporary Russia," *Culture, Medicine and Psychiatry* 24 (2000): 77–100.

Parts of Chapter 3 appeared in "Sexuality Education in Russia: Defining Pleasure and Danger for a Fledgling Democratic Society," *Social Science and Medicine* 49 (1999): 801–14.

Parts of Chapters 4, 5, and 6 appeared in "Bribes, Gifts, and Unofficial

Payments: Towards an Anthropology of Corruption in Post-Soviet Russia" in *Corruption: Anthropological Perspectives*, ed. Dieter Haller and Cris Shore (London: Pluto Press, 2005).

I follow the Library of Congress system for transliteration of Russian words, with the exception of terms that are commonly used in English and spelled differently (such as glasnost, Yulia). In cases where published references include spellings that differ from the Library of Congress system, I also retain the original transliteration of the citation.

All translations from the Russian are mine, unless otherwise indicated.

WOMEN'S HEALTH IN
POST-SOVIET RUSSIA

Introduction

CONCEPTUALIZING THE POLITICS OF INTERVENTION

"Russia has 100 Years to Live," warned the newspaper *Segodnia* in December 1998 (Derzhavina 1998). "Pediatricians Confirm That Russian Children Everywhere Are Physically and Mentally Deficient," announced another daily, *Novye Izvestiia,* in January 1999 (Malakhova 1999). In the first decade following the collapse of the Soviet Union, acute anxieties over Russia's viability as a society, a culture, and a nation pervaded that country's public discourse. Terms such as "dying out" [*vymiranie, ubyl'*] and "depopulation" [*depopulatsiia*] were standard imagery for capturing a complex series of public health and demographic processes, including below-replacement fertility levels, high male mortality, and rising rates of morbidity. Infectious diseases ranging from tuberculosis to diphtheria, cholera to syphilis, raged, some to epidemic levels.[1] Life expectancy for men plunged from 64 years to 57 between 1987 and 1994, and reached only 61 in 1998, due to causes largely associated with severe, sustained stress: trauma, alcohol poisoning, and cardiovascular disease (Vishnevskii 2000). Abortion, the major means of fertility control throughout most of the Soviet era, remained widely used; terminations reached over double the number of live births as late as 1999 (Field 1995; *Naselenie Rossii 1999* 2000).

In public commentaries and informal conversations, Russians wove images of their nation as suffering from decades of destructive socialism and the socioeconomic dislocations of market reforms. Illness touched numerous corners of daily life. And yet, anxieties over the state of society coalesced around problems of physical, social, and spiritual reproduction. Women "were afraid" or "unable" to give birth, professionals and laypersons lamented. And when they did, they and their children were said to suffer physical traumas due to years of poor health, failing health care institutions, and a polluted environment (Field 1995: 1471; Brown and

Rusinova 1997). Also to blame, many stressed, was pervasive moral decay—a problem seen as historically rooted in the population's "low level of culture" around sexual health and family relations, and exacerbated by contemporary reforms. As professionals monitored reproductive processes and designed educational projects for reproductive health, women's bodies and selves came to symbolize the unfolding destiny of a nation in demise.

Reproductive issues in former socialist states also placed high on the agendas of Western organizations with missions to advance women's equality. During these first, exhilarating years after the collapse of the Soviet Union, Western activists committed to women's rights shared a broad optimism with many Eastern European reformists about the potential benefits that democratic reform could bring. Numerous organizations ventured to provide assistance for women's issues in particular, often with little firsthand knowledge of the former Soviet world. They drew instead on arsenals of critique and decades of experience in women's activism at home, and invoked the value of gender equity to claim that portions of the multilateral and bilateral development aid for post-socialist democratization should be redirected into projects for women. Health-based organizations seized on concepts such as reproductive rights and individual choice as a way of merging humanitarian goals of improving women's health with a politically salient investment in democratic change.[2] But Western agencies often did not consider how their own knowledge was shaped by historical, cultural, and institutional experiences that post-Soviets might not share, and they rarely subjected their methods of intervention to critical scrutiny—to questions of how they, too, might be entangled in growing power relations and inequality.

I began this research in 1993 as a study of a project sponsored by the World Health Organization that aimed to promote Russian women's reproductive health, empowerment, and equity. WHO targeted maternity care as a site for reforms to improve both women's physical health and their autonomy in health care settings. Framing my inquiry as an ethnographic case study of global-local collaborations, I saw this project as offering a productive vantage point from which to observe how efforts to promote democratic reform and women's rights came together on a daily basis. For approximately twelve months between 1994 and 1995, I worked simultaneously as an independent researcher and an ethnographic consultant on Russia to WHO's Healthy Cities Project in its European Regional Branch Office. In this dual capacity as researcher and consultant, I too was seized by the optimism of this post-socialist moment, where exciting new opportunities for engaging with Russians seemed to mean an endless array of possible collaborations. My initial questions were: What did Russian women patients and Russian doctors—most of whom were also women—think about the reforms WHO advocated? How did they implement them and improvise with them in the daily work of providing maternity care? How did Russian experts and laypersons respond to WHO's rather politicized vision that recognizing women's self-determination was central to improving maternity care?

As a feminist anthropologist of Russian society, I was sympathetic to WHO's values that birthing women's voices and interests should be paramount in the delivery of childbirth services. At the same time, I also envisioned my ethnographic inquiry as itself an intervention. Culling from hundreds of hours of participant-observation fieldwork, I aimed to inform WHO affiliates about Russian health providers' and women patients' perspectives, their daily experiences, and their responses to the ongoing reforms. By ensuring that the foreign consultants became aware of any differences in cultural perspectives that separated their agendas from those of their Russian counterparts and the Russian women they were ultimately working to help, I hoped that Russians' knowledge and experiences would become central to this project's development. I believed that in-depth, ethnographic analysis into the globally led process of democratization had the potential to turn abstract concepts about feminism and human rights into effectively implemented programs in the former Soviet world. Finally, I also expected that a project like WHO's, that valued gender equity and community participation—and that welcomed in an anthropological investigator for an independent study—would be structured to address global-local equity in power and knowledge. Thus, a key question guiding my inquiry became: What could Western democracy activists and feminists learn from observing this maternity care reform process and listening to Russian voices?

My official role as a WHO consultant on this project provided me with access to St. Petersburg's maternal health care institutions, and enabled me to gather insights from both WHO and Russian experts, and birthing mothers and their families. Yet as I followed the project's process and outcomes from all their perspectives, I discovered few actual "collaborative" aspects. St. Petersburg policymakers and WHO officials had ceremoniously signed political agreements affirming the agency's values of "health for all" and community participation in health, and they shared a commitment to improving women's health as a particularly critical task. But the daily work of responding to global recommendations involved Russians in dialogues and debates that largely excluded foreigners—outsiders who, I was told, seemed to have little understanding of local experience. The WHO project thus marked the beginning of a longer trajectory my research would take that moved beyond the initial case study to explore a range of locally devised initiatives aiming to improve women's health in St. Petersburg. Accordingly, while conducting fieldwork in 1994–95 and continuing after my consultant work with WHO ended in 1996,

1998, and 2000, I expanded my fieldwork and asked a series of broader questions: What kinds of social change did pregnant and birthing patients, and Russian health care providers seek as they struggled to improve reproductive health? How were their efforts shaped by political-economic constraints of both the socialist health care system and its democratic market transitions?

Posing these questions, I found several paradoxes. Despite the WHO–St. Petersburg political agreement that expressed shared concerns for women's reproductive health, Western and Russian experts held dramatically different views on the reasons why women's health mattered and the specific problems necessary to tackle. The historical and cultural differences separating WHO and Russian knowledge quickly became evident in fieldwork and interviews. On the other hand, I also came to see that the two sides shared a set of assumptions and tactics in their disparate approaches to improving women's health. Both groups imagined that resolving the crisis in reproduction required broad transformations in Russian society. And both sides, in pursuing such changes, bypassed the structures of inequality underlying the social problems they targeted. Whether advocating for women's issues in a feminist, human-rights oriented vein or concerned with "raising the level of culture," discipline, and individual responsibility, Westerners and Russians both emphasized the need for transforming individuals' attitudes, values, and behaviors, in lieu of strengthening collective systems for human welfare.

The six cases of health interventions that this book presents are grouped into two parts: Part I, *Projects,* examines global and local health care reform projects and sex education courses. Part II, *Practices,* explores the everyday negotiations between maternity care providers and pregnant and birthing patients in maternity hospitals. In each case, we see how the effects of combining Soviet-era institutions and ideas with neoliberal ideology for democratic, market-oriented reforms led to a strikingly similar outcome: actors repeatedly dismissed the state and the public sphere as viable sources of social protection and justice. In detailing these phenomena through ethnographic "thick description," the book poses a critical challenge for feminist and rights-based activists: If projects aiming to overcome socialist-era problems are regularly displacing the responsibility for change onto *individuals,* how can public concern for *social* forms of suffering be revived?

THEORETICAL DEPARTURES

This study builds on an important body of literature concerning Russia's public health that has detailed wide-scale degradation and increasing vulnerability in all areas of social life. Such research clarifies dimensions of the post-socialist experience often disregarded in ideological images of "transition," where the breakdown of communism was initially hailed as enabling democracy, civil society, and economic revival. Qualifying such depictions, scholars have exposed the disabling effects of dismantled social safety nets, the destruction of universal, free health care, and an economic depression unknown to any country outside a declared state of war (Brown and Rusinova 1997, 2000; Caldwell 2004; Field, Kotz, and Bukhman 2000; Field and Twygg 2000; Shkolnikov, Field, and Andreev 2001). Working mainly with statistical data, interviews, and large-scale surveys, these studies have provided a fuller and more nuanced understanding of the transitions from socialism.

What remains to be done is to explore ethnographically and theoretically the ways health, and reproductive health in particular, have been sites for conceptualizing and implementing a renewed social order in Russia. Research from Eastern Europe has shown that gender and reproductive issues are central components of political-economic transformations after socialism (Gal and Kligman 2000a, b). As "democratic transitions" were announced in Poland and Hungary, for example, restrictions on abortion were immediately put forth on legislative agendas. The unification process in Germany was accompanied by attacks on the liberal access to abortion that had been available in the GDR. In these contexts, contenders for political power invoked their opposition to abortion as a sign of their ethical superiority over the widely delegitimized socialist policies (Gal 1994; Gal and Kligman 2000a, b; Maleck-Lewy and Marx Feree 2000). Only in Romania, which endured the most draconian forms of repression in the region, was the end of socialism marked with a liberalization of reproductive rights. Legal abortion ensued immediately following the assassination of Ceausescu and his wife and was viewed as a moral victory in the aftermath of severe human repression (Kligman 1998).

For liberal thinkers who assumed that intimate dimensions of life would be irrelevant to political transformations, the centrality of gender and reproductive issues to post-socialist politics appeared paradoxical. Susan Gal and Gail Kligman explain this trend by demonstrating how attention to reproduction offered East European elites moral currency for establishing a renewed legitimacy for themselves and their fledgling nation states (Gal 1994; Gal and Kligman 2000a, b; Kligman 1998). In Russia, too, nationalists have seized on reproductive issues to promote their broader political agendas. In 1992, the annual number of deaths surpassed the number of births, inaugurating what became a sustained period of population decline in Russia. The popular press and conservative academics portrayed these trends as an impending national catastrophe: the nation had started "dying out." Communist and nationalist politicians drafted bills to ban abortion, withdraw funding for family planning, and implement a range of pro-natalist policies—while presenting themselves in the process as altruistically devoted to protecting "the nation" (Rivkin-Fish 2003, 2004c). By 2003, the Ministry of Health passed the first restrictions on abortion since the Stalin era (Myers 2003). Moreover, with socialist-era pretensions of building a multiethnic society now widely discredited, pro-natalists specified that it was the size and quality of "the Russian nation" that mattered. Conservative activists emphasized that the nation's survival rested on Russian women's ability and desire to bear additional children and raise them in patriarchal nuclear families (Antonov 1995; Antonov and Sorokin 2002; Shumilin 2000).

While nationalists and Russian Orthodox activists have seized on pro-natalism and opposition to abortion, birth control, and sex education as means of establishing their political legitimacy, it is paradoxical that those actors striving to improve health at the local, clinical level have largely dismissed collective action as a viable means of change. This is particularly notable given the recent emergence of women's activism in other sites and for other issues in Russia (Hemment 2000, 2004; Kay 2000; Sperling 1999).[3] One midwife I met, Lena, who left the maternity hospital system after thirteen years to work semi-legally in homebirths, articulated this view most succinctly: "I guess that some global transformations, global reforms are bound to happen in Russia. But you must change yourself, not the system but yourself. If you change yourself, everything around you will change, people will become kinder [*dobree*] . . . to change yourself is to change inside, your inner nature. . . . It's a question of inner freedom, it's beyond the government structure" (Rivkin-Fish 2004a).[4]

Though Lena's decision to leave the official hospital system was unusual, her views on the necessary approach to social change were strikingly common. Many Russians' strategies for healing themselves and their society strove for moral transitions in persons, such as new attitudes and behaviors and renewed expressions of care and connection in interpersonal relations. To be sure, these moral shifts addressed the deployment of power and the redistribution of status and authority, sometimes aiming to eradicate and sometimes to maintain forms of domination in daily life. But even as they set about to re-create state-citizen relations in the spaces of public health clinics, they evaded official, governmental sources of power, avoided collective, social interests, and resisted making claims in the name of broader societal needs. They considered improving health and morality to be possible without politicized collective activity, for they viewed the revival of spiritual, ethical, healthy selves as incompatible with aspirations for political power. Rather than engaging oneself with official state spheres and struggling for influence over policymaking, efforts to improve health involved disassociating oneself from arenas marked as "official," working informally to cope with constraints generated by the state, and locating "transition" in one's own attitudes, behaviors, and commitments.

At the same time, global and state policies introduced innovations in health services that endorsed similar modes of change, which I conceptualize as "individualizing" or "privatizing." While Russian policymakers celebrated the ideological dimensions of reforms aiming to stimulate moral kinds of change such as increased individual responsibility, neoliberal reforms left people increasingly vulnerable socially and economically, and failed to address systemic forms of disempowerment inherited from the Soviet system. In effect, neoliberalism lent further credence to long-standing views of politics as "dirty," tainted, and unfeasible as a mode of genuine social change, while furthering Russians' experiences of disenfranchisement.

The fact that women patients, doctors, and other professionals consciously delegitimized state authority in the health care setting makes their projects and practices especially relevant for understanding post-socialist change. The chapters in this book explore several of them. I begin with the global health project affiliated with WHO. This case study traces what happened when ideals about the need to politicize health and expand women's rights were put into practice as concrete goals of an international development project. Achieving "women's self-determination in birth" became primarily an obligation of individual health care providers, who were to create "democratic" change through adopting new attitudes and behaviors with women patients. Chapter 2 examines the neoliberal arguments of Russian health care planners that financial incentives to "stimulate" doctors would be the key to improving Russian health care. Aiming for change at the level of providers' values and behaviors through mechanistic, individualizing solutions, these policies ignored the collective, systemic disempowerment of health care workers in political-economic and gendered ways. Chapter 3 explores Russian sex education work, innovative projects for health promotion in which medical practitioners also placed all the hope—and burden—for improved health on individuals. They neither advocated public policies, nor lobbied for increased resources, nor invoked critical arguments about state policies when teaching children and teenagers about health needs. In Part II, we see the strategies that women patients and doctors devised to ensure healthy pregnancies and births. In chapters based on ethnographic narrative and analysis, I highlight the multiple kinds of formal and informal approaches people used to deal with changing but systemic forms of constraint. In both free state services and newly emerging fee-for-service contexts, women patients and doctors relied on themselves and personal networks of friends to overcome poverty, bureaucracy, and abusive forms of power in pursuit of healthy reproduction.

A central ethnographic finding of this study is the continual under-mining of thinking about collective needs and collective forms of action in the post-Soviet era. But it is necessary to understand that these trends did not lead actors to deny or debate the widely circulating political discourses about the vulnerability of one particular imagined collectivity—"the Russian nation." This study illuminates the ways state and nationalist interests became at once ignored and inscribed in the health promotion work of institutions and the daily practices of experts and citizens. In global efforts to further a post-Soviet "transition," too, rhetorical claims for improving the public health and working for community empowerment sat side-by-side with reform proposals that neglected collective modes of action and societal forms of responsibility. In the process, such projects rendered the structural violence privatization wrought on the state health care system and its workers invisible.

The approach used in this study is based on the conviction that attempts to study and intervene in women's health in the former socialist world (and indeed, women's and men's health anywhere) involve the deployment of power. In a context where global interventions are intended simultaneously to be health-enhancing and empowering for marginalized groups, acknowledging the role of power and inequality in interventions implies a further task: the need for global activists, international consultants, and the organizations that sponsor them to restructure their methods and objectives to reflect the democratic commitments they profess. The anthropological methods of research I employed aimed simultaneously to understand global activism and local realities on their own terms and also to consider how Western projects for democracy and women's interests might better translate feminist insights about empowering social change in *locally* meaningfully ways.

These concerns to make sense of the politics of intervention for democratic change parallel broader trends in studies of Eastern European societies to rethink the concept of transition and its imagery of linear, evolutionary change as a paradigm for capturing post-socialist processes. [5] Moving beyond a teleological vision of the transformations occurring since the fall of socialism, scholars have increasingly analyzed the contested values people assert in establishing a sense of newness, difference, progress, or loss, as they face increasingly stratified opportunities and pressures. These questions, furthermore, have opened up a burgeoning concern with the ways changes after socialism are being created at the site of personal identities, life strategies, and subjectivities. Of particular interest is how neoliberal policies and the constraints of a global economy have demanded new ways of situating bodies in space and time, and reorienting and disciplining selves. [6]

Closely connected with these issues is the problem of how post-socialist changes reconfigure the division of society into public and private spheres, a process with direct implications for gender relations, norms of femininity and masculinity, and women's and men's opportunities. I draw on Gal and Kligman's (2000a) semiotic approach to understanding "public" and "private," viewing these concepts as discursive distinctions constructed and contested in daily practice, rather than as fixed realms in society associated with concrete spaces or spheres of activity. This approach calls attention to the ways that "public" and "private" may be "nested" inside each other—such that under socialism, the home became split into valued, "public" activities in which politics was debated and planned, and "private," invisible activities such as women's domestic labor (2000a: 49–54). Daily interactions in the medical workplace were similarly split into official duties and unofficial or personalized practices, such that doctors at one and the same time saw themselves as officially responsible for providing competent care to all patients, and unofficially responsible for providing a different quality of attention to those patients with personal contacts among the staff. Understanding the various changing forms of such practices opens up inquiry into the ways power and inequality are being made invisible, or taken as "natural," as socialism is both actively dismantled and increasingly forgotten.

"Public" and "private" are not the sole conceptual units dividing social life into distinct spheres of activity, each with its corresponding ethical demands for responsibility and reciprocity. In tracing the strategies for social change weaving throughout the health care sphere, I came to see three distinguishable types of action that divide persons from society at large, the state, or the public. For analytical purposes, I categorize them as individualizing, personalizing, and privatizing strategies.

Individualizing strategies are primarily two approaches to creating social change. First are the numerous educational projects aiming to develop people's personality [*lichnost'*] and its related components, such as new attitudes and behaviors. These may be devised by experts in a pedagogic frame, such as for moral education [*vospitanie*] on health, hygiene, and sexuality; or they might be the planned outcome of health system reforms designed by experts seeking positive consequences of market reforms at the level of individual health providers' behaviors. In both these cases, the individualizing strategies are "official" or "formal" in that they are publicly announced and intended for universal appropriation.

The second kind of individualizing practices are devised by persons in their daily life as a self-imposed form of discipline aiming to create social change. The best example here is when the midwife Lena says, "You must change yourself, not the system but yourself. If you change yourself, everything around you will change." I consider such practices informal because they emerged in the context of daily life, particularly during conversations about social change, rather than during formal projects by officials announcing what social change should look like. They are not "unofficial," however, in that they do not serve as resistance to official dictates or mandates (an aspect central to personalizing strategies).

Personalizing strategies of change stem from the Russian cultural practice of recognizing certain persons as "our people," those who embody the potential for trust, mutual understanding, and reciprocity [*svoi liudi*]. This is an inherently moral concept that is implicitly opposed to bureaucratic sources of contact, power, and authoritative knowledge. I speak of personalizing strategies in ethnographic contexts when doctors and patients strive to transform the public, bureaucratic character of the health care setting by personalizing it—replacing official, standardized protocols with the obligations and interactions of kinship and friendship. Such strategies tend to differ from individualizing practices in that they are embedded in and reconfirm certain types of interpersonal relations, rather than assuming people to be individual islands unto themselves. An implication of this is that personalizing strategies also tend to represent unofficial kinds of practices, since they evade institutional procedures, legal rules, and officially recognized forms of authority. I stress here, however, that personalizing strategies must not be summarily dismissed as instances of "corruption," for they are often perceived by participants to be evidence of higher moral activity than many official practices. When based in acquaintance relationships and friendship bonds, these strategies are exclusionary.

Privatizing strategies of change are global and state policies that seek to privatize formerly public services, such as in the creation of fee-for-service health care and a consumer model of the patient role. These are official and formal in that they are the subject of governmental policy. However, fee-for-service care is also occurring in informal and unofficial ways alongside the official framework. When doctors and patients negotiate fee-for-service care in a way that suits them better than the official procedures, they are strategizing for privatized kinds of change in an informal way. It is possible that in the future these privatizing strategies may increasingly subsume personalizing strategies among some groups, if economic forms of relationship become more acceptable and a personal basis for relationships seems less necessary or desirable. In the context of this study, the key difference is that personalizing strategies draw on the emotional and moral element of personal relations [*svoi*], whereas in privatizing strategies, the utilitarian element of business/monetary exchange is overt and legitimate.

It is not surprising that creating forms of "privacy" has been a central part of the first decade of post-socialist reforms. Economic privatization, of course, is a key element of market reforms, and the notion of a "private" sphere unencumbered by state interventions is integral to the vision of liberalism advanced by democratizing organizations working in former socialist societies. At another level, however, it is not at all self-evident that democratizing reforms intended to pluralize the means of communication, forms of ownership, methods of economic exchange, and life courses of citizens would need to be carried out in socially exclusionary, *privatized ways.* That is, why have democratic reforms focused on disciplining individual attitudes and behaviors while re-creating institutional procedures and economic forms to benefit only a few? In shining a spotlight on these paths of change, I suggest that we must critically question why recent efforts to improve Russian women's health have re-created oppositions between formal and informal interests and reinstated the value of personal as opposed to collective needs, distinctions that were so central to life under state socialism.

ON NEW REGIMES AND NEW PERSONS

Many of the strategies of change that I refer to as individualizing, personalizing, and privatizing have historical roots. The Soviet project established imperatives for people to cultivate new attitudes and behaviors appropriate to a collectivist society. Leaders of the Bolshevik Revolution expected that people in the new revolutionary order would come to display the characteristics of a socialist personality, distinguished by a commitment to the tasks of collective life and building communism. The need to cultivate that personality type, however, was not to delay the revolution itself. Marxist-Leninist ideology held that human beings are shaped above all by the material conditions of their environment, so early Bolshevik leaders prioritized the transformation of social conditions as the prerequisite that would enable further psychological and moral changes. Still, the eradication of private property and reorganization of economic relations did not automatically lead the proletariat to assume a proper socialist consciousness.

The new revolutionary society endured the devastating effects of civil war, famine, the Nazi invasion and the consequent war, tragedies that left millions dead and, in the eyes of the regime, hindered the complete realization of socialist transformation. In the early 1950s Stalin elaborated a theoretical explanation for the stubborn resistance of "vestiges" [*otstatki*], the psychological tendencies and behaviors "left over" from the former bourgeois regime. Building on and adapting Marxist theory, he argued that changes in the superstructure followed a dynamic partially independent of economic relations (de George 1969: 5). Developing a socialist personality therefore required special tactics aimed at cultivating a new form of social consciousness. Socialist moral education would become an instrument for state planners and professionals to deploy in the struggles against crime, alcoholism, and other forms of "anti-social behavior."

Oleg Kharkhordin has argued that the Stalinist regime placed concerted emphasis on constructing and disciplining a specific kind of individual, one whose ritualized performances of self-fashioning would serve the interests of the Soviet state. Thus, while "individualism" is often opposed to policies of collectivism (in capitalist as well as Soviet rhetoric), a certain vision of the individual [*lichnost'*] nonetheless became a depository for moral demands made of Soviet citizens (1999). These demands included self-sacrifice, heroism, and steadfast loyalty to the revolutionary cause through unwavering convictions and unhesitating actions (Sinyavsky 1990). On the domestic front, individuals were also to embody particular forms of modernization and discipline. An important tool for shaping these dimensions of the new personality was the concept of *kul'turnost'*, or "culturedness." *Kul'turnost'* is based on the pre-revolutionary Russian aristocratic notion of *kul'tura* [high culture], which evokes knowledge of the canonical texts of Russian literature and the high levels of spirituality they symbolize. Stalin drew on the enormous symbolic capital of *kul'tura* to promote discipline and conformity to images associated with civilized high society, progress, and modernity. Being "cultured" came to mean having both erudition in classical literature and art and competency in social etiquette, a combination of personal qualities supposedly antithetical to vulgarity, cruelty, and evil (Boym 1994; Dunham 1990 [1976]; Volkov 2000). Despite these positive associations, *kul'turnost'* has also been used to signify class, race, and cultural difference, serving as a weapon of power and exclusion (Lemon 2000).

Reproductive politics was another key arena where Soviet experts worked to change individual values and behaviors, rather than expand economic resources for well-being and ensure political empowerment. Beginning in the late 1960s, demographers raised extensive concerns about the continuing decreases in fertility in European parts of the Soviet Union. Although some fertility specialists explained low fertility by citing poor material conditions and women's difficulties combining the double burden of full-time paid labor and housework, other prominent specialists portrayed urban women as selfishly rejecting family life in favor of consumerist values. Their policy recommendations aimed to celebrate the importance of home life and re-instill the maternal instinct, considered to have been diluted by socialist policies of women's full employment (Antonov 1986; Kvasha 1981). State policymakers listened: it was certainly cheaper and easier to generate messages about family values than to resolve housing shortages and invest in childcare resources—the obstacles to higher fertility identified by competing specialists.[17] So-called sex-role socialization courses were instituted in high schools to ensure that young women prioritized marriage and children and that all young adults embraced traditional stereotypes about women and men's distinct psychologies and social roles (Attwood 1990). In popular media and scholarly writing, sociologists and other specialists attacked the "one-child family mentality" considered rampant among educated and professional sectors (Antonov 1982; Antonov and Medkov 1987). Significantly, while few part-time opportunities or other improved conditions for women's employment materialized, the one systemic kind of welfare reform that was established involved extended maternity leaves. Images of women as mothers and nurturers, rather than as workers, came to dominate media representations of women (Posadskaia 1992). Such depictions were not coincidental: they often explicitly aimed to reverse earlier Bolshevik experiments to create New Soviet women as equal to (now disparaged as "the same as") men, and to revive the "natural" association between femininity and maternity. Despite these discourses, fertility rates continued to fall.

The fact that Russian women and men did not comply with state pronatalist campaigns should serve as a cautious reminder against assumptions that Soviet ideology was an all-powerful force acting on people's worldviews and behaviors. But it is also notable that in evading state pronouncements, people turned to strategies based in ideas of a personal sphere. In economic areas, too, Russians regularly strategized during the Soviet era to obtain scarce goods by positing a realm of personal, as opposed to collective or state, interests (Ledeneva 1998). The recreation of such informal strategies as a means of obtaining trustworthy, competent health care is examined in Chapters 5 and 6. Here, it is important to note that since the postwar period, many women and men came to believe that focusing on the family offered an alternative to investing in the state and collective interests. The Russian writer Tatyana Tolstaya, critiquing American feminist perspectives that view women as individuals with interests apart from their family, has called the family in Russia a centrally important "moral refuge" from the state (Tolstaya 1990; see also Funk and Mueller 1993). Efforts to improve women's health sought to protect that "moral refuge" from perceived attack by invigorating people's commitments to it.

In Chapter 3, we will see how lectures reconfirmed the notion that a personal sphere existed opposed to politics and insulated from state ideology. Educators sought to protect family life from harmful taboos about sex created under the Soviet era, and from perceived dangers of chaotic sexuality in the post-Soviet marketplace. Lectures presented formulas for achieving harmonious marriages and emphasized that healthy social change would be a product of individuals working on themselves. Gynecologists lectured on women's needs to postpone sexual activity and avoid abortion by introducing religious discourses constructing the fetus as a "child" and abortion as the "sin" of "murder"—discourses that opposed Soviet atheism, materialism, and legal abortion. Psychologists sought to change young people's attitudes toward sexuality and their intimate practices by attacking Soviet ideology on sexuality. Their lectures aimed to encourage students to appreciate sexuality as a central part of human nature and marriage. Thus, while physician-educators did not actively promote childbearing for the sake of national vitality (as many politicians and demographers did), neither did they challenge demographic discourses that claimed a serious fertility crisis existed, nor did they suggest that debate on childbearing might be reoriented to make political demands for social welfare. The strategy of promoting sexual health through inspiring moral changes in individuals' attitudes and behaviors seemed the most promising and legitimate tactic educators could employ. It built on historical methods of social change, and in a context of continuing distrust of the state and public (market) spheres, this approach put medical expertise to work for the goal of strengthening traditional families.

METHODS

On an August morning in 1994, a white-coated midwife with a starched blue hat stood in the middle of the hall of the hospital's prenatal ward and shouted, "Everyone come to a talk!" Within a few minutes, thirty-some pregnant women poured into the ward's lounge, leaving behind the rooms they shared with one, two, or three others. The women had on their own nightgowns and slippers, but the flowered robes that they had all been issued by the hospital to wear on top of their nightgowns created a kind of patient uniform, and indeed made them appear a uniform mass. I sat among them in the white coat that Dr. Natalia Borisovna, chief of the ward, had instructed me to wear each day I came to conduct fieldwork. Facing her patients, Natalia Borisovna set out to inform them of a whole host of changes, from the hospital's new birthing procedures to its revised recommendations for infant care. She began by explaining that this maternity hospital was working in accordance with the World Health Organization project called "Healthy Cities," and to make that connection seem real, she pointed to me, saying, "Michele is a representative of the WHO."

"What does this [affiliation with WHO] mean? Today in St. Petersburg only 1 percent of all newborn babies are healthy. I mean totally healthy, and here we're working for healthy babies. This is not to say that all of your babies are going to be sick, but there may be small things, allergic reactions, for example, so now we're trying to do things a bit differently."

She continued by explaining that in accordance with WHO recommendations, the hospital now had individual delivery rooms, allowed companions during labor and visitors during scheduled hours, and housed babies together with their mothers to encourage feeding on demand. Swaddling babies was no longer acceptable, and, in the attempt to encourage breastfeeding, hospital staff would no longer give pacifiers or bottles. She warned the women that their own mothers were likely to tell them to swaddle or give the baby supplements and that they would need to inform their husbands that they should only breastfeed. She then spoke at length about the importance of breastfeeding for the baby, urged women to get good nutrition while nursing, and with a large dose of humor, tried to disabuse them of the myths surrounding breastfeeding:

"Young women sometimes think, 'I won't nurse, because I want my breasts to be beautiful and nursing will ruin them.' Let me tell you, once you decide to keep the pregnancy . . . then your breasts are already going to change. If you're like me, and your chest is a size –1 [0 is the smallest Russian size. —MRF] then when you're pregnant, you'll get up to about 5 (laughter), then later they'll shrink back, as before. So nursing won't make the difference; once you're pregnant, that's that."

A woman in the audience raised her hand and asked, "What is the ideal length of time for nursing a baby?"

Natalia Borisovna glanced at me and stated, "Well, we say six months is about right, a year is the optimum, the maximum. Isn't that right, Michele?"

Taken somewhat by surprise, I intuitively strove to confirm Natalia Borisovna's words, and said, "Yes, about a year." But I felt uneasy being called on for "expert" confirmation. I was neither a medical doctor nor a public health specialist. It was through mere serendipity that, while traveling to St. Petersburg in 1993 to conduct preliminary research into Russian women's health, I met a senior official from WHO's Copenhagen-based office on the airplane. We found it amusing and intriguing that we shared common goals for going to St. Petersburg, and he invited me to participate in a conference sponsored by WHO's European Regional Branch that he was about to co-host in the historical Russian city. The conference focused on the Healthy Cities Project, a program that the UN-based agency promoted as a resource for urban planners, activists, and citizens dedicated to revitalizing public health policies. The St. Petersburg municipal government had recently joined the program and was establishing its own Healthy Cities Project with an emphasis on improving reproductive health. Six months or so later, I presented this official with a proposal to conduct an independent study of the Healthy Cities Project underway in St. Petersburg. He accepted my proposal, agreed that I would set my own research agenda, and gave me the title of "temporary consultant" to WHO's Healthy Cities Project to help me gain access to relevant city institutions.[7] We both hoped the insights I provided would be helpful in improving the project's success.

By the time I sat in that hospital lounge, I knew that the WHO experts working with St. Petersburg were avid proponents of breastfeeding for the first year or more, and clearly Natalia Borisovna agreed with their recommendations on this issue. Yet I wasn't sure what breastfeeding meant to these women, how they planned to feed their babies, or what challenges women would face with different approaches.[8] Moreover, while Natalia Borisovna's urgings on breastfeeding followed WHO's recommendations, they also seemed to contradict the agency's other messages about promoting women's self-determination and autonomous decision-making in health care. In my mind, the foremost task was to learn how women and their providers understood WHO's recommendations, not to advocate for particular behavioral changes without knowing the cultural and political-economic context of reform.

In reflecting back on this moment some time later, I realized that Natalia Borisovna's cue for me to confirm her advice reflected several important issues relevant to the ethics of my research and role in Russia: First, as a foreigner and a representative of the WHO, I had a degree of authority to speak about health-related issues, despite the fact that I personally had no expertise on these matters. Moreover, as I conducted fieldwork in this and other health care institutions, this authority could be appropriated to support Russian physicians' claims to pregnant women. I would thus need to conscientiously detail exactly what the purpose of my presence there was, what my knowledge base consisted of, and to whom my recommendations (if any) would be targeted, to each person I met. In explaining my links with WHO, I took pains to explain that I was advising the agency about the cultural and political specificities of Russia, not evaluating local compliance with agency recommendations. I saw value in many of WHO's suggestions, but rather than asserting they should be implemented locally, I was investigating whether Russians were promoting these suggestions, as well as how they were doing so or why they were not.

If I partially sought to distance myself from WHO by clarifying my role as an anthropologist of Russia, I did not want to disassociate myself from the agency: I felt that my link with WHO could be beneficial in inducing Russians to share their views on health and health reforms with me, since I hoped to be able to influence agency policy and project development. I kept this hope at the forefront of my fieldwork for twelve months in 1994–95, when I lived in St. Petersburg and conducted daily fieldwork in maternity hospitals, women's outpatient health clinics, the city's Public Health Committee, and the homes of people I met in these sites. Yet in the course of that year, as affiliates of WHO's Healthy Cities Project came to St. Petersburg to promote reforms in women's health, I realized that the agency had no mechanism for incorporating cultural knowledge such as I was providing into the project design. While the insights I offered about the workings of local clinics were greeted with interest, there was no clear way to transform them into practical action. As earlier scholars had found when examining development in the Third World, adding anthropological insights alone would have little effect on people's health and well-being outside of broader structural changes in agencies' work (Escobar 1995; Ferguson 1994; Justice 1986; Morgan 1993). Even while using the language of "community participation," "political will," and "women's rights," development agencies had not substantially reconfigured their methods for stimulating change. I became further committed to producing a cultural and political analysis of local efforts to improve Russians' health, in part as a means of critically assessing the possible roles of global activists in projects for post-socialist change. A key concern inspiring this book is to promote a self-reflexive concern with the use of power in feminist-inspired projects (Rivkin-Fish 2004b).

Throughout my seven years of research I renewed relationships formed earlier and also became acquainted with a range of people situated in different locations in the health care arena. While in St. Petersburg, I spent time with women patients and medical personnel, health policymakers, physicians (obstetricians, gynecologists, pediatricians, general practitioners [*terapevti*], and anesthesiologists), and midwives, nurses, hospital administrators, and housekeeping staff. I observed the interactions between Russian physicians and patients during prenatal exams and admitting interviews, during childbirth, and in the postnatal wards. I met with women patients in their hospital rooms, often on the prenatal ward as they rested under observation for a pregnancy at risk or waited in the last days of pregnancy for labor to begin.[9] I sat in on lectures that gynecologists, obstetricians, and psychologists gave to women for sex education and childbirth preparation, and by showing interest in their work, got to know many of these providers well. I conducted fieldwork during retraining programs for Russian health professionals conducted by both WHO affiliates and local medical experts, and visited sites where home birth midwives, working outside the formal public health system, conducted prenatal visits and childbirth and parenting preparation classes.

Official institutional spheres were not the sole contexts for fieldwork: applying the anthropological practice of cultural immersion, my research also involved living with Russian families and participating in the lives of my informants outside the narrow confines of the health care institutions. Through the hospitality and curiosity of hundreds of Russian women and men, I shared in the daily activities of patients, health care providers, and their families who agreed to discuss their experiences of managing their health and their lives in the first decade of the post-Soviet era. At times I was invited to their homes for a meal or tea, a formal interview or an informal chat; sometimes I hosted new acquaintances myself. With still others, I talked about women's health in city parks, museums, and the numerous palaces of Russia's former aristocracy.

My commitment to participant-observation as a methodology led me to approach women patients, providers, and other Russians first and foremost by expressing my interest in learning about their perspectives on women's health and the social changes connected with the end of the Soviet era. Anthropological analyses of interviewing as a methodological strategy have noted potential problems with this "speech event," which led me to treat interviews cautiously and with a certain degree of improvisation. An interview is an artifice from the point of view of conventional modes of communication in daily life. It introduces a rupture in the normal flow of life that can inhibit, rather than advance, outsiders' understanding of local knowledge and the logic of people's practices (Briggs 1986). To deal with these issues, I employed a variety of strategies for learning in the field. In meeting women on prenatal (or sometimes postnatal) wards, I rarely began by seeking out individual women or providers for formal interviews. Instead, I undertook "participant conversations," in which I joined groups of women and providers in their ongoing discussions, explained my research agenda, and sought permission to raise questions related to my research. This approach provided me with insights into a range of issues connected to local strategies for improving women's health, broadened my sense of the social worlds of the hospital, and allowed me to identify people who would be amenable to participating in one-on-one interviews and even ongoing social relationships with me.[10] From these encounters and through additional acquaintanceships, I conducted more in-depth interviews, lasting between one-and-a half and three hours, with women, providers, and policymakers. Again, however, my method focused more on developing intimate relationships and contextualizing the insights I was gaining in terms of people's lives than on acquiring large numbers of one-time interviews based on little interpersonal trust. To make contact with women from the highest socioeconomic classes who had accessed paid services, I employed a Russian research assistant with extensive networks among these groups. Finally, continued, in-depth discussions and frequent correspondences became possible as some Russian friends gained access to email and a few were able to visit me at home in the U.S. The WHO project that initially inspired this research thus became the starting point for numerous sets of inquiries regarding Russian health care and global and local strategies of change beginning in 1993 and continuing through 2000. My fieldwork and the friendships it spawned enabled me to share in the lives of ordinary citizens and professionals through their pregnancies, births, and sometimes deaths, their marriages and divorces, new jobs, and the mundane, daily stuff of their survival.

POST-SOVIET HEALTH AND THE ANTHROPOLOGY OF MEDICINE

At the beginning of their collaboration, WHO and Russian public health experts identified the high rate of maternal mortality in St. Petersburg (over 60 per 100,000 live births) as a key dilemma characterizing women's reproductive health.[11] Both sides recognized that social and cultural conditions, not only biological factors, were at work. WHO highlighted the medicalized character of care, which viewed pregnant women as ill and requiring continual medical surveillance and subordination to health care institutions, as contributing to poor health outcomes. Russian experts insisted that women's "low level of culture," high rate of abortions, and low compliance with medical authority were largely to blame. These competing explanations confirm basic anthropological insights that health, disease, and healing cannot be grasped by examining biological factors alone.[12] Still, the spate of epidemiological studies emerging over the last decade on former Soviet people has paid minimal attention to the ways that personal experiences of sickness, and the social relations that organize healing, become meaningful. Nor have most scholars connected socioeconomic processes of disintegration and change after socialism with the changing meanings of health, disease, and healing. Adriana Petryna's (2002) study of "biological citizenship" after Chernobyl presents an inspiring exception. She demonstrates how the scientific and bureaucratic institutions serving officially recognized Chernobyl "sufferers" have shaped the construction of Ukrainian selves as ill and disabled, a necessary survival strategy amidst widening impoverishment and despair (2002). Petryna and other anthropologists examining communities around the world that have endured ongoing violence and loss emphasize the integral relationships between biological illness and "social suffering."[13] At some levels, public health scholarship has worked to incorporate social and political-economic dimensions into its analyses: WHO's own definition of health recognizes it as "a state of complete physical, mental and social well-being and not merely the absence of disease or infirmity." But it has not incorporated an anthropological sensitivity to the diverse meanings and experiences associated with "well-being" and "disease" in particular communities. As a result, such research often cannot capture the historically situated logics through which ordinary people strategize for health—ideals and practices that diverge widely within and across societies.

For example, a central thread in Russian culture considers individual, "spiritual" suffering to be not only common, but virtuous, a sign that one's life is motivated by his or her conscience (Pesman 2000; Ries 1997). And while the physical degeneration read into the country's public health indicators has been presented as a different, national experience of pain, the abiding concern with spiritual dimensions of interpersonal relations was never far removed. Poor health and low fertility were portrayed as the accumulated outcome of a spiritual morass in which individuals lost the guidance of their conscience, *failed to suffer,* and actively or passively enabled a degenerate system to forge degenerate persons (Pravda.ru 2003). Russian projects and practices for women's health built on moral imperatives of interpersonal accountability and combined them with both Soviet discourses celebrating expert authority and neoliberal assertions about personal responsibility. In this way, the pursuit of "well-being" constituted processes of reproduction in the broadest possible sense, the labor of giving life to symbols, values, and practices of identity in a newly marketized world.

MEDICALIZATION IN THEORY AND ETHNOGRAPHY

This ethnography of efforts to improve Russian women's health also contributes insights to the analysis of knowledge/power in biomedicine, a field of inquiry known as the study of medicalization. Since the 1970s, discourses and practices of biomedicine have been a fruitful arena for analyzing the changing nature of power in modern societies. Although critical studies of medicalization can trace their roots to Marx (Illich 1976; Navarro 1977), an important inspiration for the study of biomedicine came from Michel Foucault (1973, 1980). Foucault argued that overt forms of repression by the sovereign had characterized political orders in Europe until the eighteenth century, but the advent of liberal democracies transformed the ways power would be exerted. As they proclaimed the disappearance of power through discourses of freedom and rights, these regimes generated new conditions for power relations to emerge, less visible and less perceptible forms for them to assume. The creation and use of authoritative knowledge became a central form of discipline and control. Both the individual body and the body of society became important sites where knowledge/power became deployed—not by states alone, but by a range of experts and institutions seeking standardization, normalization, and order. Foucault termed the knowledge/power derived from the discipline and control of individual and social bodies, such as their life cycles and reproductive processes, *biopower.* Biopower became the goal of regimes and experts as they assumed the right and responsibility for measuring, monitoring, and intervening to improve both "the population," and individual persons in the name of societal good, including health and welfare. For example, expert discourses often took the "self" as an object of prescriptions regarding "normal" ways of acting, so that caring for "the self" in appropriate ways became the responsibility of modern citizens. Exertions of biopower thereby came to be accepted as beneficial and necessary, rather than as coercion (Foucault 1980, 1988; Lock and Kaufert 1998; Lupton 1995; Petersen and Bunton 1997).

Medical knowledge and practice are among the foremost expressions of biopower in contemporary society. When particular behaviors or conditions become designated as "problems" in a biological or medical sense, or when suffering becomes recognized as a matter for health providers to diagnose and treat, these conditions become medicalized. Once labeled in this way, they become considered phenomena of "nature," as opposed to manifestations of "God," social forces, or political inequalities (Lock and Kaufert 1998: 17–18). A critical issue that scholars of biomedicine have addressed is that medicalization—with its diagnostic focus on biological processes and its therapeutic mode of curing individuals, of locating pathology at the site of the body and the self—displaces attention from the power relations inherent in medical care. Political-economic and social causes of suffering are ignored, made invisible, or left outside the realm of potential redress. Medicalization negates or brackets out the effects of social context and domination, while presenting itself as a humanitarian, objective, neutral purveyor of objective truth, neither affected by social and cultural processes nor implicated in regimes of power. Politics goes unrecognized in medical diagnoses and efforts to repair bodily and social ills (Lock and Kaufert 1998: 20).

Critical observers of Russia interested in documenting medicalization can find ample cases in which experts and institutions worked to normalize individual bodies, and used disciplinary techniques to measure, monitor, and intervene in women's lives and reproduction. WHO consultants, for example, identified numerous techniques used to control Russian women and transform their childbearing experiences into pathologies requiring medical interventions. But ironically, the consultants' critique of the medicalization of birth derived from a universalizing view of professional power that failed to capture the complex inequalities of socialist and post-socialist health care. Their suggested reforms for maternity care were founded on a caricature of medical practice, as one consultant explained to me— "doctors everywhere want to keep the power for themselves." Yet precisely what kind of power did Russian doctors have? Unlike physicians in the West, they were deeply impoverished, often earning considerably less than their patients. Providers confronted this perceived injustice regularly, as in Nina Petrovna's rueful comment, "We walk home from work on foot, while they [patients] pass us in their Mercedes," and in patients' supercilious attempts to pay doctors to do extra work or even undertake orderlies' labor, such as bringing them bedpans. In addition, doctors enjoyed an extremely limited scope of autonomy in the daily workplace. They were impotent to affect the fractured system of pregnancy and childbirth services that they knew impaired patient care and powerless even to determine their own work conditions and schedules. The subordination doctors experienced took its toll on a daily basis, for their voices and interests were ignored at all levels of the health care bureaucracy.

My fieldwork experiences helped me see that the complex practices occurring in hospital encounters cannot be captured by the analytic of medicalization alone. In addition to the unfamiliar constraints on physician power, it is notable that Russian patients frequently did not construe medical power and technological interventions to be benign or benevolent, and they often questioned the necessity of experts' prescriptions. As a consequence the clinic setting was fraught with animosity and distrust of medical power. At the same time, no simple binary opposition between powerful doctors and victimized patients can adequately capture these relationships. My field notes are filled with stories of patients' and doctors' strategic maneuvers to achieve a responsible, respected form of professional expertise. And as I developed close relationships with both women patients and hospital staff, I came to see that power, domination, inequality, and disenfranchisement traversed multiple and contradictory channels—even when the structure of relations in the clinic clearly favored medical expertise.

As I confronted these issues, the process of narrating clinical encounters between doctors and patients became a profound challenge for me, one that brought long-standing scholarly discussions on the ethics of representation vibrantly alive (e.g., Fine, Weis, Weseen, and Wong 2000). Writing about provider-patient conflicts in a way that solely highlighted doctors' techniques of discipline and domination filled me with unease: this approach did not do justice to the lived realities and systemic constraints I had seen in the clinic, and seemed a betrayal of the complexities

I had been entrusted to understand. My close friend Karina, who had worked as a housecleaner in a maternity hospital where I conducted field-work, offered me important advice for dealing with this dilemma: "You must include in your book the words of B.G. [Russian poet and folksinger Boris Grebenschikov], 'Everything I do is an attempt to live like a human being in conditions that are inhumane,'" she wrote me in 2003. This comment captured the pathos of hospital conflicts perfectly, and guided my writing. It reminded me to orient my analysis around the ways that systemic constraints of unending poverty and bureaucratic abuse shaped the search for dignity, respect, and morality. Theoretically, it helped underscore the imperative for a historical, political-economic, and cultural analysis of physician power.

My approach to the issue of medicalization has thus sought to move beyond the mere documentation of particular disciplinary techniques and processes. I use medicalization as the starting point for an inquiry into how Russian doctors and patients distinguished between appropriate and abusive expressions of professional power, and strategized in particular ways to create "benevolent" forms of expert power (see also Lock and Kaufert 1998). I explore how their understandings were linked to broader visions of Soviet and post-Soviet societal ills and how people's knowledge of ethical forms of provider power were changing. I have focused my analysis on demonstrating the particular contradictions that made doctors committed to medicalized forms of authority, uncovering subtleties in the ways different health providers deployed expert knowledge/power, and detailing the multiple forms of systemic subordination that women faced and strove to overcome as both users and providers of health care services.

NEGOTIATING SOCIALIST MEDICALIZATION

A key point is that Russian women's strategies for negotiating medical power drew on their broader cultural knowledge of Soviet bureaucratic power. The Soviet health care system epitomized the institutional apparatuses of socialist state power, which, as Katherine Verdery (1996) has demonstrated, undertook the functions of rule in fundamentally different ways than capitalist states did. In accordance with the principles of central planning rather than markets, the purpose of socialism was to accumulate the means of production rather than profits or surplus value; the state's power resided in its ability to accumulate resources and maintain control over their distribution. In this way, Verdery suggests (1996: 19–57), the socialist state seized citizens' time, disciplined their bodies, and ensured their dependency. Socialist regimes, moreover, worked in both repressive and productive ways. On the one hand, they engaged in surveillance, prohibition, and the repression of dissent, while on the other, they sought legitimacy through paternalistic redistribution. The realm of health care exemplified these dynamics, and the ideology of medicalization gave them further momentum. The medicalization of citizens' health allowed state experts to monopolize the means of production and maintain control over the distribution of social products (in this case, health services), and it offered a conceptual framework for justifying both repressive and productive forms of power. At the same time, the Soviet state worked to limit professionals' power, too. These dynamics emerged in institutional and individual levels of practice, in the organization of birth control, abortion, and childbirth. I describe these briefly below, and explore them further throughout this book.

Shortly after assuming power in 1917, the Bolshevik regime instituted a universal and free system of health care. Until the Soviet Union's demise, Party leaders cited the achievements of their health care system as evidence of their commitment to citizens' welfare. Yet for neither patients nor providers were the conditions in which treatment took place satisfactory. Without denying that the Soviet health care system realized certain important gains, such as universal coverage, one may also argue that the system's greatest achievement was the power it delivered to the state. In reproductive health, for example, free abortions were available to women on demand up to twelve weeks and for "social reasons" through the second trimester. Yet contraceptive supplies were in continual deficit, neither produced domestically nor imported in sufficient quantities. Condoms were of poor quality and never promoted by the public health authorities, while methods such as diaphragms and spermicide were virtually nonexistent. Oral contraceptives were briefly introduced in the 1970s but were quickly removed from distribution networks due to the unpleasant side effects of high-dose hormones. The state committed no resources to their further research and development. In the late 1980s, the IUD was the most widely used among what are considered "modern" methods of birth control, used by approximately 12 percent of adult women surveyed in the Soviet Union (Remennick 1991). Most others relied on techniques such as the rhythm method, calendar method, and douching, and resorted to the frequent use of abortion when these methods failed. The heavy reliance on abortion was perfectly suited to the logic of state socialism, for it facilitated the state's control over the most effective resource for limiting birth. It also ensured the greatest degree of medicalization of women's bodies: with few methods of preventing pregnancy available, state experts maintained a monopoly over the legal means for women to intervene and interrupt unwanted pregnancies.

The medicalization of childbirth achieved similar outcomes. Women

were characterized as ill, in need of expert control and technological interventions at all phases of pregnancy and birth. Prenatal care was separated
from childbirth services, eliminating continuity of care throughout pregnancy and birth. In the maternity hospital, mothers were separated from
their babies, feedings were scheduled according to institutional regimes,
no visitors were allowed, and no companions for women were admitted
during labor. Women were kept in maternity hospitals for five days following vaginal births and for seven days following caesarean sections if
no complications arose. Health providers were socialized with the ideology that women patients know little about their bodies and their health
needs and should submit obediently to the dictates of health professionals.
Courses in preparation for childbirth, for example, concentrated on "teaching women how to behave properly" during birth rather than ensuring
that they understood the processes of labor and delivery and empowering
them to participate in decisions about medical interventions. Here we see
the closest similarities between Soviet and Western medicalization.[14] However, the power physicians derived from the two systems of medicalized
maternity care differed immensely.

Discursively, the Soviet state (like its Western counterparts) celebrated
the authority of technical elites, including doctors, and encouraged public
compliance with expert prescriptions. But the Bolsheviks eliminated physicians' corporate power by disallowing independent medical associations.
In Western countries, such associations play a central role in consolidating
the political-economic influence of professions, by representing and promoting members' interests to the state, market forces, and the public. Prior
to the Bolshevik Revolution, pre-revolutionary medical associations, including Russia's most powerful, the Pirogov Society, had been active in
social debates and expressed criticism of both the czarist regime and the
Bolsheviks. Yet the new Communist leadership was intolerant of competing social forces, and dissolved these associations. The Communist Party
became the sole channel through which physicians could impact government policies regarding their work-related interests (Field 1991: 47–48).
Moreover, the Soviet state undermined the class basis of physicians' power.
Doctors were paid according to wage scales set by central planners, at rates
below those of manual laborers. This political-economic disenfranchisement has been described as the deprofessionalization of medicine. It transformed physicians from politically empowered corporate agents, actively
negotiating their interests, into workers with a status structurally analogous to bureaucrats, who were subordinated to the vertical hierarchy of
the state system. Even as late as the last years of the Soviet regime, Mark
Field argued for the "political nonexistence of the Soviet medical profession" (Field 1991: 48).

There were gendered dimensions of this process. An estimated 70 percent of Soviet physicians were women, with even higher proportions in the fields of obstetrics and gynecology. The Soviet state recruited women into medicine, but then treated the field as less valuable than masculinized occupations such as engineering, which were perceived as directly contributing to the so-called productive spheres. Given these layers of constraint and relatively limited prestige, Soviet doctors occupied a significantly more constrained form of elite status than did doctors in Western liberal settings. As Field has noted, the clinic setting became the primary site for physicians' exertion of professional dominance (1991: 53). The ideology of medicalization gave health care providers the one form of social dominance they would have under the Soviet regime: the symbolic power of expertise.

And still, the authority to wield this power often remained elusive for physicians; to the extent that patients considered physicians' power to derive from the state system, their legitimacy as healers was in question. In this way, the health care sphere exemplified the bigger problems of legitimacy that plagued the entire Soviet system: the actual benefits the paternalistic state offered fell far short of the promises it made to provide humane and liberating entitlements. In Verdery's felicitous phrasing, "The lived experience of people in socialism precluded its utopian discourse from becoming hegemonic—precluded, that is, the softening of coercion with consent" (Verdery 1996: 23). For example, although medical care was readily available, women resented the bureaucratic inconveniences and obstacles to obtaining care that they routinely faced. They often encountered physicians who seemed indifferent, their skills and motivations dulled by a system that did not reward initiative and diligence. The institutional inconveniences, poor accommodations, and seemingly apathetic providers led many women to describe health care settings through images of factories, such as "a meat grinder" [*miasorubka*] or a "conveyor belt" [*konveor*], where they would be treated mechanistically and their individual needs, concerns, and comfort ignored. And when the state withdrew from welfare provisioning following the demise of the Soviet regime, what remained of public services drastically deteriorated. Ordinary women (and their male partners) thus confronted health care institutions with widespread distrust during pregnancy and birth. Their challenge to the legitimacy of health providers' endeavors did not express a critique of relations based on expert domination per se; nor was their reluctance to trust physicians generally based on doubts about science as a mode of knowledge or source of truths. It emerged out of the contradictions between the state's ideology of providing humanitarian care and the women's practical experiences, rumors they heard, and expectations they developed of indifferent, incompetent, and uncaring treatment provided in health care institutions. It was the association between expertise and state bureaucratic power that rendered medical authority and professional domination highly suspect in Russia.

When the state's monopoly on social services began unraveling during Perestroika and after the Soviet Union's collapse, new ideological and institutional forces came to shape the reproductive health industry. Economic reforms had a substantial impact here. "Free" health care services suffered from collapsing budgets and deficits of necessary supplies, while providers' salaries were infamously insufficient to support a family. On the other hand, local clinics and hospitals were given the option to become self-financing [*khozrashchetnye*] and to offer fee-for-service care for elective procedures such as abortions and for luxury accommodations or nontraditional care during childbirth. Yet with diminishing state regulation and no nongovernmental organizations devoted to protecting health users' interests, even women with financial means were unable to exert much control over the procedures undertaken during birth. Many still faced the prospect of entering a state institution with a frightening sense of vulnerability. To obtain competent reproductive health care and protect themselves from abusive exertions of state power, women deployed a variety of strategies for relating to providers, which I document ethnographically in Part II. They spoke of "taking responsibility for themselves" by seeking information about the birth process, or rejecting the prescriptions of physicians they did not trust, or trying to negotiate better care from providers on an informal or formal basis. But under the expansion of market reforms and governmental decentralization, both the means women could deploy to avoid official power and the ethical character of the privatized, personalized worlds being created were shifting. Women's various methods for overcoming the vulnerability and victimization often endured in state institutions offer examples of how new forms of stratification and class difference are coming to shape everyday practices in post-socialist society. Yet women's individualizing strategies usually failed to blunt the coercive aspects of medicalization, which remained ideologically and institutionally integrated into the health care system even as it underwent reforms touted as enhancing "consumer choice."

Russian women's experiences of medicalization thus differed from those of many women in the West, in part because they regularly felt the need to contest and negotiate the ways medical power would be deployed. Russians' distrust of medical power reflected culturally specific logics, critiques of the injustices of state domination. Stated otherwise, because ordinary citizens had a language for conceptualizing and critiquing the domination they experienced at the hands of state bureaucratic power, medical authority—a form of state power—was not automatically rendered legitimate. Women associated it with the incompetent, ineffective social service system that did not prioritize (or often meet) their needs. In this way, they shared an assumption with many providers, who recognized that structural constraints related to socialist bureaucracy—forces glossed colloquially as "our system"—formed the root of daily obstacles.[15] Yet although both laypersons and experts identified the collective, institutional framework of constraint when speaking of "our system," they also located that system's most tangible effects in the behaviors and attitudes of those they conflicted with in the clinic. With very few channels of addressing structural problems, their solutions largely focused on transforming persons and interpersonal relations—privatizing strategies that usually left systemic constraints untouched. In birth, many women were left feeling emotionally betrayed and physically violated.

STRUGGLES FOR AUTHORITATIVE POWER

Doctors' strategies of disciplining individuals and interpersonal relations offer important insights into the ways medicalization occurred in socialist and post-socialist contexts. They also reveal how informal practices that had been common during socialist times persisted and changed under post-Soviet conditions. During fieldwork in a state maternity hospital between 1994 and 1995, I found that doctors regularly disassociated themselves from state power to establish their integrity as professionals. This was not a ploy for personal material gain. Doctors yearned for respect and legitimacy as healers, but confronted the frustrating dilemma that as human embodiments of the state system, they were greeted with widespread public mistrust. Doctors themselves felt robbed by the poverty and bureaucratic rigidity of "our system." These constraints impeded them from being fully competent in delivering medical care, and in turn left them without the respect they felt they deserved. The main solution— short of leaving the health care system altogether—entailed symbolically separating themselves from the negative aspects of the system in everyday practice. They did so in many ways: by lamenting the "collective irresponsibility" structured into the health care system; by insisting on taking "personal responsibility" for their work, often against official rules and in spite of the personal risks that unsanctioned actions involved; and by creating informal social circles with other providers and some patients that acted as emotional buffers against the dominant institutional framework. Strategies of personalizing the public, official sphere of power at once enacted a kind of resistance to it and reproduced it, by redirecting privileges to ever tightening social circles, rather than totally subverting it.

Physicians' construction of a professional identity in opposition to "our system" was thus particularly fraught and ironic. As their informal tactics symbolically separated them from the illegitimate state and its capricious bureaucracy, doctors did not acknowledge that they, too, represented that system and had partial access to its power. To make sense of this process, I borrow the term "misrecognition" from Bourdieu (1977, 1990, 1994). I argue that providers' desperate desire to experience themselves as authoritative, influential, and respected experts led them to naturalize (and thus legitimize) their dominance over patients. In this way, providers misrecognized their own techniques of controlling patients by considering these strategies to be qualitatively different from the abusive actions of other state bureaucrats that they encountered and resented. Providers' use of the concept of "our system" as a shifting signifier illustrates how this misrecognition operated. In daily conversations, doctors referred to "our system" to mean a variety of things: its referent might be the fragmented, bureaucratized health care system at one moment, the aggressive reproaches of their superiors at another, and the apparent ignorance and indifference of women patients (attitudes seen as mirroring broader state policies toward health), at the next. The phrase "our system" did not refer to a physical place or particular public setting. Rather, it captured aspects of constraint associated with state power by which providers felt victimized, professionally and personally, on a daily basis. No one ever used "our system" in reference to themselves. If doctors, as employees of the state, could misrecognize their own power to such an extent as to construct patients as empowered adversaries while asserting their own victimization, it is clear that there was no objective boundary between participants in "our system" and the moral community for informal relations; there were no objective criteria for designating empowered groups in this logic. The elusive need to achieve—and be acknowledged as achieving—ethical forms of caretaking and control mobilized physicians' battles and alliances with patients, policymakers, and protocols.

It is important to recognize that physicians' sense of victimization, and their intense discomfort with being a part of "our system," was exacerbated by several factors in the mid 1990s. Conditions in the state health care system had substantially deteriorated and showed no signs of improvement. On a daily basis, this meant that clinics and hospitals regularly had no hot water and that their infrastructures stood crumbling with no hope of repair, while hospital medical staff were required to undertake housekeeping and maintenance work such as landscaping and the cleanup after a flood. Much of physicians' time was spent figuring out how to protect and carefully distribute the meager supplies of medicines that were supposed to be provided by the state to all patients for free. Despite policymakers' rhetorical concerns about raising fertility, they were neglecting and abandoning women's health and had left most doctors "on the front lines" of the reproductive health crisis alone. In this context of betrayal and despair, physicians saw themselves not as representatives of "state power," but as disempowered medical experts left to deal with the fallout of indifferent state planners—specifically, the high rates of maternal morbidity that complicated the births they attended.[16]

In many cases, doctors deployed individualizing solutions to excise people or relationships from the warped spiritual clenches of "our system." Generally, such maneuvers involved extending hierarchical forms of control over patients yet further. For example, providers' tactics included frequent attempts to promote "personal responsibility" among their patients through what Bourdieu (1977: 189–90) calls "crude" ways of deploying expert authority: yelling, chiding, and berating women patients and didactically demanding "responsibility" from them. In other cases, providers strove to personalize the bureaucratic sphere by working with patients on the basis of kinship and friendship obligations. These informal frameworks granted providers the possibility of transcending their symbolic association with the state system as they reached out to women patients—and were treated in return—as *svoi liudi*, our people. Yet the constant threat that these strategies would be reframed by others as "corruption" or "bribery" tainted many of these efforts with risk, and limited the degree to which such practices seemed liberating for providers. In most of these cases, too, hierarchy, exclusion, and systemic constraints continued to plague doctors' and women's struggles. Chapters 4, 5, and 6 explore ethnographically the complex dynamics through which providers and patients sought to achieve key values of human interactions in Russia—care, concern, commitment, responsibility, accountability, conscience, competence, and *kul'tura*— through formal and informal strategies of negotiation. Repeatedly, we see the ways in which providers tried to disassociate themselves from hospitals' bureaucratic power, which they themselves experienced as oppressive and constraining, but ended up misrecognizing that they, too partook of its domination over women. I show that such processes of dissociating oneself from "our system," along with efforts to change patients, constituted strategies of "transition" away from socialism as a moral process lodged in oneself and others, but inadvertently reproduced socialism's core contradiction of collective disenfranchisement.

Few informal exchange relations entirely overcame the ongoing structural problems of the health care sphere. Even with the establishment of legal, paid services in the maternity system, which would ostensibly preclude the need for contacting an acquaintance to obtain quality health care, many women found that their needs and interests were still not prioritized. Women's (and health planners') assumptions that improved health care could be achieved by stimulating individual providers with financial incentives failed to ensure consumer guarantees and protections against incompetent care or medicalized domination. Again, though ideologically palatable, overcoming socialist power through interventions targeted at personal attitudes and behaviors fell short of resolving problems of a systemic nature, such as patients' lack of political-economic and legal protections and health workers' deprofessionalization and socioeconomic disenfranchisement.

Western observers tended to assume that the advent of democratic reform in the former USSR would enable authentic civic expression for ordinary people and professionals, ending the need for the pervasive deception and subversion of official systems assumed necessary for survival under the Communist Party-State. Any lingering reliance on informal processes and procedures, it was thought, could only reflect intrinsic Russian failures—cultural tendencies of deceit, or an inbred disrespect for the rule of law. This study counters such assumptions through ethnographic inquiry into daily negotiations of the health care sphere. It argues that many everyday strategies for overcoming systemic inadequacies strove to realize ethically sound tactics in interpersonal relations (even if this involved misrecognizing one's own complicity in power). As the new constraints of market democracy became increasingly visible to many Russian people, they gave up believing that the necessary amounts of public resources would be allotted to keep welfare services functioning or that legislative acts would actually ensure citizens' rights. Ironically, changes made in the name of "democracy" and "liberalization" after the Cold War have generated and justified indifference to the plight of social needs and have left actors to rely on *private* strategies to compensate for such indifference. Russians have turned to informal personal networks, drawn on private resources of all kinds, and worked to remake *themselves*.

In the conclusion to this book, I consider what the focus on changing individual attitudes, behaviors, and morals as a means of improving women's health suggests about post-Soviet change more generally in Russia. The strategies of individualizing, personalizing, and privatizing changes for improving women's health raise enormous challenges for feminists committed to reducing social inequities based in gender, class, and ethnicity. I argue that it may be possible to reconfigure feminist initiatives to work more effectively in post-socialist contexts without abandoning these core values. Promoting the empowerment of women, the poor, and the marginalized first and foremost demands self-reflexive attention to our own methods of conceptualizing problems and working for change.

PART 1
Projects

ONE

Promoting Democracy through Moral Correction

"For me, it's a universal right, and it's that simple. No woman should be forced to have anything shoved inside her against her will. It's as true and universal a principle to me as are child labor laws."

Susan Jones, a North American midwife consulting with the European Regional Branch of the World Health Organization, accompanied me on a walk through the streets of downtown St. Petersburg one evening in the early months of 1995.[1] Our conversation began when I mentioned that as part of my research on Russian women's health, I wanted to understand what brought her to St. Petersburg, and how she was trying to accomplish her goals. Her impassioned response referred to a clinical practice she and her colleagues were trying to eradicate in Russian obstetrical care—the routine use of enemas at the start of women's labor. This procedure, once common in Western maternity care, too, was used to empty the bowels prior to childbirth, and thereby ensure against defecation during pushing and the potential infection of the baby. In the 1970s, advocates within the US women's health movement scientifically refuted the notion that enemas lowered the risk of infection. Moreover, they reinterpreted the routine use of this procedure as one example of many hospital interventions that served a primarily symbolic function: making birth a medical event in which women were to be subordinate to scientific authorities and expert power (Boston Women's Collective 1999; Davis-Floyd 1992).

For this midwife and her team of consultants in Russia, ending the compulsory use of enemas represented a broader set of convictions that women have rights to self-determination, humane treatment, and choice about medical interventions in childbirth. By conjuring up the humiliating, violent image of women "having things forcibly shoved inside" them, Susan characterized the broader system of Russian reproductive health care as dehumanized, and in need of drastic reform along democratic principles of treatment. In her capacity as a midwifery activist for eighteen years in North America and India, Susan had dedicated her professional life to protecting women against the abuses and cruelty that occur when the needs of an institution, and not the individual, are given primacy in health care. Similarly, her current work in Russia aimed to bring this sensitivity about women's individual needs for choice to the staff of local reproductive health services.

Susan and her colleagues associated with WHO worked to carry out reforms in St. Petersburg in the mid-1990s to promote women's health and well-being and connect them conceptually with democratization. The story of efforts to "democratize" Russian maternity care offers a case study of how the logic of Western development assistance was extended in the mid 1990s to rebuild former socialist societies. As Western organizations sought to transfer assistance and expertise to the former Soviet Union as a means of building democracy, the kinds of solutions often proposed—from the need to build civil society to protecting women's reproductive rights—aimed to empower citizens (Hemment 2000, 2004; Rivkin-Fish 2000, 2004b). Attention to women's rights enabled important issues to enter Russian public discourse in new ways, even if the outcomes of projects differed from their planned objectives (Hemment 2004). At the same time, assistance projects also became an important site for articulating interpretations of the end of the Cold War as the triumph of liberal democracy over state socialism. As Western experts embarked on the process of promoting democracy and women's rights, they may have missed the chance to explore how power, domination, and justice lined up differently in the (post-)socialist context. The unwavering confidence in "true and universal principles" that Susan asserted had the unintended effect of sidelining the ethical and methodological dimensions of inducing change. But we need to ask: How can our methods of promoting democracy reflect the values we strive to convey?

WHO and St. Petersburg forged links just after the fall of the Soviet regime. The project to reform maternity care was undertaken by a delegation of experts who were affiliated with WHO but were not full-time employees of the agency.[2] Their work had been preceded and enabled by a direct connection that the WHO's European Regional Branch undertook in St. Petersburg in the early to mid 1990s. With hopes high that democratic freedoms would soon proliferate throughout Europe, WHO officials in Copenhagen invited the St. Petersburg city government to join the Healthy Cities Project, an international network of municipalities working to improve urban health. Becoming a member of the WHO-coordinated network required displays of "political will" by municipal officials in the form of independent action to promote health and equity: they were expected to commit economic resources to a defined arena of public health

problems and promote the development of multi-sectoral cooperation between the state, community groups, and the private sector for health goals.
These objectives represented clear attempts by the international agency to
have local governments address the political and economic dimensions of
health. By inviting St. Petersburg leaders to join the Healthy Cities Project,
WHO officials saw themselves as promoting a social and political agenda
for change, in which the ideals of democracy and equality would shape
health interventions.

However, with a maternal mortality rate estimated to be ten times
higher in St. Petersburg than in the UK, WHO officials felt that admission to the Healthy Cities Project network must not be the only kind of
engagement undertaken with the Russian city.[3] Development assistance,
they believed, was also important. The connections forged through St.
Petersburg's Healthy Cities Project would facilitate further projects, including ones structured to provide advice to an ailing, needy country.

I focus on two stages of maternal health projects that followed this
initial agreement in St. Petersburg: (1) a Consensus Conference held early
in the collaboration that was documented in agency reports; (2) an educational workshop that consultants held in the spring of 1995, which I
observed. Despite the ease with which the two sides agreed to focus on
maternal health, the significance they attributed to the issue differed dramatically. I describe the divergent agendas that St. Petersburg officials and
consultants affiliated with WHO brought to their collaboration, differences that only became clear to participants as the project evolved. Then,
drawing on anthropological critiques of development, I show how the
methods of "consensus building" and educational training for democracy
worked selectively to highlight inequalities in interpersonal interactions,
while leaving the structural bases of disempowerment invisible and intact.
Consultants did not recognize the contradictions of their intervention,
however. Their profound commitment to the critique of medicalized birth,
coupled with their acceptance of the systemic limits of development work,
cut short any doubts. They approached the process of catalyzing change
without inquiring how the unique social and political-economic conditions of women's health care under state socialism might have created distinct problems and methodological challenges.

COMING IN FROM THE COLD (WAR):
A RAPPROCHEMENT IN 1992

Hope and enthusiasm inspired WHO officials as they reached out to
invite St. Petersburg to join their network of Western European cities in
the Healthy Cities Project. On the heels of the Soviet Union's collapse,

Western organizations and agencies were eager to use their experiences and know-how to help shape the kind of democracy Russia would become. Becoming a "Healthy City" required municipal officials to create policies that reflected WHO's conception of health as "not merely the absence of disease, but a complete state of physical, mental, and social well-being" (Alma Ata 1978). As city policymakers prioritized the agency's goal of "health for all" by addressing problems of unequal access and the specific needs of marginalized groups, active involvement in the Healthy Cities Project would pay off for St. Petersburg, as it gained international recognition as a leader in public health. The projects St. Petersburg supported would become the subjects of discussion and observation abroad, and Russian public health officials, nongovernmental organizations (NGOs), and ordinary citizens would have opportunities to meet with and learn from their counterparts working on similar public health projects throughout Europe. Although the Healthy Cities Project was not a direct source of financial support, the exposure and status gained as a WHO "Healthy City" carried the promise of helping the city forge additional connections throughout Europe that might lead to economic and technical support. In both Healthy Cities literature and personal statements by WHO officials, the project appeared to directly engage the political process by requiring states to reduce inequality as a key to improving public health.

This blueprint for political action rested upon the ability of WHO officials to find (or nurture) willing partners among Russian policymakers, so-called political will. For St. Petersburg's leaders, collaborating with the international agency was promising but also risky: it required exposing the inadequacies and vulnerabilities of their system after decades of Soviet secrecy regarding public health. The rapprochement between St. Petersburg and WHO began with a formal acknowledgement that the city's maternal mortality rate approximated 70 per 100,000 live births, ten times higher than in Western Europe (Stephenson and Porter 1994: 2). St. Petersburg officials embarked on their Healthy Cities Project by designating four institutions that would serve as models for reform throughout the city: a maternity hospital would transform women's and infants' care along WHO recommendations for a "Baby-Friendly Hospital"; a major city abortion clinic had recently been transformed into a center for family planning and reproductive health; a comprehensive center for teenage reproductive health had been founded; and a fourth center for teen mothers was planned. These centers were held up by city officials as evidence of their city's commitment to the Healthy Cities Project and dedication to improving maternal health. The commitment to equality would be realized through providing entitlements for vulnerable and impoverished sectors of society to obtain prenatal and postnatal consultations at the Baby-

Friendly Hospital, as well as free contraceptive supplies. Homeless women would have the opportunity to receive free room and board in the Baby-Friendly Hospital for up to twenty-one days after giving birth, during which time they would be assisted to find alternative housing. WHO saw these pilot programs as promising beginnings to what it hoped would become a widespread reform process throughout the city. However, municipal officials developed no concrete plans for creating community involvement or multi-sectoral action in such projects, and as time went on officials did virtually nothing to expand their scope. Although serious questions soon emerged regarding St. Petersburg's commitment to the Healthy Cities Project, WHO officials remained committed to working in the former Soviet city, which, it was felt, sorely needed public health care reforms.

MATERNAL HEALTH AND HISTORICAL CONSCIOUSNESS

The decision to prioritize maternal health deserves examination, for what appeared at the time to be a straightforward agreement based on mutual understanding obscured two distinct sets of concerns about women and the necessary roles of the public health system. For Russian experts, maternal health was an area of great societal importance because it is directly linked to the reproduction of the nation (Rivkin-Fish 2003). Although Russia's low birth rate had been the subject of political concern since the late 1960s, further declines in fertility and sudden, rapid increases in mortality and morbidity following the collapse of the Soviet Union in 1991 augmented Russians' anxieties about their nation's vitality and future. Journalists and politicians from throughout the political spectrum regularly cited demographic and public health indicators as ominous signs of the nation's present and future vulnerability (e.g., *Delovoi Peterburg* 2000; Gridasova 1994; *Novaia Gazeta* 1999; Semenov 1996). Communist and nationalist politicians and journalists went the furthest, directly blaming market economics and Western-style reforms for the country's ruin (Khorev 1995, 1997; Medvedeva and Shishova 2000).

A general consensus in Russia held that improved economic conditions and political stability would be necessary prerequisites for improved public health and fertility rates. Physicians tended to blame the severe poverty and social crisis for the breakdowns in women's health, including sky-rocketing rates of STDs, kidney disease, and anemia. They also described poor reproductive health indicators as a symptom of "our women's low level of culture," by which they meant Russian women's putative ignorance and apathy about healthy behaviors. In considering how Western aid could help them manage the crisis, doctors hastened to emphasize their own capabilities in scientific, technical, and manual skills and mainly highlighted their need for medical technology. It was the *deficit* of medical technologies, from basics such as disposable gloves, needles, and antibiotics, to sophisticated equipment, not the value of technologies per se, that physicians considered the main problem. While welcoming WHO experts as a source of material assistance and even an exchange of information about clinical techniques, Russian experts dreaded the possibility of being didactically instructed as members of a backward, underdeveloped nation.

As WHO consultants on maternal health investigated St. Petersburg's situation, they interpreted the city's problems in dramatically different ways. Birth rates were of minimal concern. Even maternal mortality, the ostensible reason that assistance was needed, was only one of three issues consultants outlined in addressing women's health and well-being. As negotiations for St. Petersburg's entry into the Healthy Cities Project were underway, consultants issued a report identifying the specific areas of maternal health care they thought it necessary to address, including not only "an extremely high and rising maternal mortality rate which is both abortion and obstetric related," but also the "severely dehumanized nature of services and older regulations preventing possible change" (WHO 1993b: 4).[4] The latter concerns referred to a range of procedures that thoroughly medicalized the childbirth process. Hospitals made routine use of interventions in childbirth—such as enemas, pubic shaving, and episiotomies—that in the West have been found scientifically to have no medical benefit. Labor and delivery took place in large wards, with several women giving birth at the same time. Afterward, women were separated from their infants, who were kept in nurseries and brought to their mothers' rooms for scheduled feedings. The hospital also isolated women from their families, by prohibiting both companions during labor and visits from relatives in the days after birth. Women had virtually no choice about their labor and delivery experiences, hospital procedures, or infant care. The entire organization of maternity care functioned to subordinate the mother-child relationship to the medical institution's needs for convenience and professional dominance.

In citing the "dehumanized" nature of services and obsolete regulations, WHO consultants laid the groundwork for future intervention that went beyond bringing St. Petersburg into the Healthy Cities Project. The global agency would support projects targeting caregiving ideologies and the provider-patient relationship during birth. Consultants called for new provider attitudes toward birth, including the recognition of patient "choice" in birth procedures, as necessary to the "democratization" of Russian health care services.

These recommendations reflected a prominent series of public health ideals that had been circulating throughout Western Europe and parts of North America since the 1970s. Members of the delegation to St. Petersburg were devoted activists who had fought for these changes in maternity care in their home settings for decades. As middle-class, educated professionals, they countered widely held public beliefs in physician authority with a view of women as the authorities on their own health needs. They advocated for policies that fulfilled people's basic social and economic needs, rather than relying on high-tech equipment and interventions. They also lobbied for broader changes in traditional public health approaches, emphasizing that community participation in health policies, individual choice, and empowerment were central to well-being (Bunton and Macdonald 1992). The work of these and related groups soon bore fruit, for in grassroots organizations and academic scholarship, and eventually in WHO policies themselves, a social model of health became an increasingly prominent alternative to the curative, medical model, with its reliance on biomedical expertise and technology (Alma Ata 1978).[5] In the mid 1980s, advocates of this social model of health succeeded in making their ideals central to WHO's policies on maternity care. WHO launched a campaign aiming to reform maternity care worldwide on the basis of these principles. The WHO Report on Health Promotion and Birth (Wagner 1994b: 361–78), issued in this context, stated:

> Childbearing issues involve fundamental human and civil rights, which should be inviolable. Specifically, these are women's rights to: complete information regarding all aspects of care, both self-care and health and medical care options; choice of place of birth, as well as of caregiver and birth attendants, including supportive friends and/or relatives; privacy during all care giving activities; choice about which, if any, interventions to accept; experience birth as a highly personal, sexual, family event; sustain the mother-child relationship throughout the post-birth period, without fear of separation.
>
> We urge all governmental and private bodies concerned with human rights in all countries to include an examination of the conditions under which childbearing takes place as one index of any nation's, or indigenous people's, civil and human rights. The WHO asserts its intention to locate autonomy, authority, and the definition of need in the childbearing woman and her family, and in their community, rather than in the professional community or in the state. (Wagner 1994b: 363–64)

WHO's Healthy Cities Project similarly defined the pursuit of social well-being through individual and community empowerment as an obligation of government. It encouraged societal recognition of the importance of individual choice to health and well-being. When the opportunity arose to collaborate in St. Petersburg, WHO consultants were eager to link the causes of women's rights and self-determination with the spirit of democracy that they believed had emerged in countries of the former Soviet Union. They defined the institutional acceptance of women's rights to autonomy in childbirth as a measure of democratic reform. Russia's problems, in this logic, at once stemmed from the absence of democratic traditions and reflected universal trends of professional dominance and the misuse of technologies. Privately, consultants admitted that these ideals were far from achieved in Western contexts, too, but they did not emphasize this fact while interacting with local Russians.

The striking differences in historical experience and cultural knowledge that WHO and Russian experts brought to their collaboration were not made explicit when the two sides initially made their agreement. The focus on maternal mortality, based in the seemingly objective language of public health statistics, reinforced a sense of shared expertise and mutual understanding about the problems needing attention. But the formal agreement effectively masked the fact that Russian experts saw the maternal health crisis as an issue of low fertility, related to government-created poverty, technological deficits, and women's apathy, while WHO consultants understood the matter of political-economic commitments to have been addressed, and viewed the ongoing professional disregard for women's rights and autonomy as continuing problems. Even as the consultants gradually encountered conflicting assumptions in the course of their country visits and meetings, they rarely sought to investigate the reasons behind particular perspectives that Russians held. Language barriers and time constraints made sustained dialogue seem too difficult; and the existence of a signed agreement seemed to preclude its necessity (Rivkin-Fish 2004b). Thus, consultants pressed ahead with a project to promote reforms in Russian maternity care by changing providers' ideologies of care. They devised an educational training workshop targeting Russian health providers' attitudes and behaviors about women's needs in birth as the primary method for stimulating reform.

A DEVELOPMENT AGENDA FOR POST-SOVIET CHANGE

Anthropological research has documented how the development industry's widespread inattention to cultural knowledge has stymied many projects' abilities to achieve humanitarian goals (Justice 1986; Sobo 1995; Stone 1986). In health-related work, scholars have demonstrated the importance of incorporating a community's conceptions about the sources of illness and health into project designs and the necessity of engaging seriously with indigenous methods of healing in order for changes to be considered meaningful and desirable among those targeted for assistance. But cultural differences between donors and recipients are not the greatest obstacle to achieving improvements in local community well-being. Recent scholarship has focused on the paradigms of knowledge and techniques of intervention through which development organizations define problems in the local context and devise solutions for their improvement. Focusing specifically on the delivery of aid to former Soviet and socialist countries, anthropologists have exposed how many development consultants and NGO/foundation officers entered into projects with rigid, bureaucratized modes of operation and with no awareness of local conditions (Abramson 1999; Hemment 2000, 2004; Wedel 2001). Wedel (2001) showed how the Western strategy of developing personal relations with a few select elites as a way of building understanding and "trust" created a series of international "clans" that directly facilitated the large-scale corruption and expropriation of resources intended for humanitarian work and development.

Theoretical analyses of development that build on Foucauldian perspectives help explain why it is that projects repeatedly fail to achieve their goals of relieving suffering and improving well-being. In his studies on madness, crime, and sexuality, Foucault's method of inquiry sought to understand how and why certain things were brought together, examined, and spotlighted as relevant to mental illness, crime, sex (and personhood), while other things were omitted as irrelevant. Foucault posed the issue thus: "what are the elements which are relevant for a given 'problematization'?" (quoted in Lemke 2000: 8). In turn, scholars examining development work have taken on his approach to examine the process of "problematization" in a given project—to ask why and how certain issues, but not others, become targeted for change by development interventions. James Ferguson (1994), for example, demonstrated how development planners rely on a series of discursive regularities as they propose solutions to ill health, poverty, and suffering. These discourses reflect the principle of governmentality—a view that "the main features of economy and society must be within the control of a neutral, unitary, and effective national government, and thus responsive to planners' blueprints" (Ferguson 1994: 72). Working with assumptions of governmentality, therefore, systematically leads development planners to designate certain kinds of phenomena as relevant problems and to devise specific types of solutions to resolve them. Development projects offer technical inputs, such as building dams, opening markets, and improving infrastructures, to alleviate poverty. Such solutions are favored because they appear to be apolitical, neutral, and universally applicable methods of facilitating improved standards of living (Escobar 1995; Ferguson 1994). The state becomes treated as the medium for implementing the changes, but never as the source of poverty itself. In addition, problems that emanate from forces beyond the state (such as the interests of foreign capital) or that involve internal political struggles (such as the interests of one political party against another), or those with no readily addressable solution (such as the complex political-economic legacies of colonialism), become considered superfluous and are omitted from development discourse, since these kinds of problems cannot be addressed within the development framework. Yet in bracketing out these relevant political forces and treating the state as a neutral mechanism for delivering social services, development projects cannot effectively address the causes of poverty, disease, and underdevelopment.

At first glance, WHO's work in St. Petersburg seemed to be distinct from conventional development projects. The Healthy Cities Project required demonstrations of "political will" and commitments to resources for health. Instead of offering technological inputs for improving birth outcomes, WHO's recommendations targeted the *misuse* of technologies and the medicalized approach to care during birth as preeminently political issues—violations of women's human rights. Yet if WHO's project highlighted the important issue of women's power as health care users, it addressed this issue only in the narrow context of interpersonal relations vis-à-vis health care providers, rather than as the outcome of precise political-economic structures that shaped provider-patient relations, such as health care users' lack of collective power and provider deprofessionalization (also a gendered issue).[6] Indeed, after securing the city's agreement to prioritize health, WHO consultants narrowed the scope of their interventions to changing the attitudes of front-line providers. The presentation of necessary attitudes and models of interpersonal interaction became a new kind of "technical input" as development agencies expanded beyond their conventional project areas in the developing world to the industrialized, highly literate region of Eastern Europe. And upon realizing that St. Petersburg officials had not followed through on many of their commitments to the Healthy Cities Project, consultants felt unable to take the municipal government to task for their neglect. When city officials undertook no community outreach to elicit and fulfill health care users' and providers' needs, and there were no consumer groups or provider associations sufficiently organized to articulate those needs and to demand that they be met, WHO consultants did not strive to enforce the requirements for community participation and political-economic investments that were embedded in their own Healthy Cities Project criteria. Instead, global experts took the city government's stated commitments to health, made to gain membership in the Healthy Cities Project, at face value. They did not investigate how the city's concomitant health care policies had exacerbated conditions of poverty, contributed to ill health, and forged new barriers to the provision of competent health care services. In line with the assumptions of governmentality, the WHO-sponsored project treated state and municipal officials as neutral agents delivering services, and removed them from the arena of potential critique and intervention. Achieving "women's rights" in birth became the responsibility of health providers alone.

CONSENSUS-BUILDING AS A DEMOCRATIZING STRATEGY

I was not involved with WHO at the early stages of its project in St. Petersburg, so my discussion draws on the agency's documentation of its work at the time. What is evident is that consultants felt a significant amount of ambivalence regarding the stance they should take while collaborating with their Russian colleagues. On the one hand, maternal health indicators were dire enough to suggest that local officials did not possess the knowledge and skills needed to effect positive change, and consultants were inclined to establish a mentoring sort of relationship with Russian public health experts. On the other hand, the Healthy Cities Project represented itself as a framework of action where democratic forms of engagement for health were an explicit goal. Governmental bodies were to collaborate in innovative ways with all levels of community representatives to bring about citizen empowerment and improved health. As one WHO official explained to me, the overtly hierarchical overtones of a mentoring relationship did not seem an appropriate strategy for approaching St. Petersburg colleagues. These competing values regarding which stance to adopt did not, however, become the subject of reflexive analysis among global consultants. They played out in rather unconscious ways in the agency's written documents and personal interactions in Russia.

These contradictions were reflected in the agency's report on the 1992 Consensus Conference on maternal health care, issued at the time St. Petersburg's involvement in the Healthy Cities Project was taking shape and given to me when I became involved in the project in 1994. This document works explicitly to construct a portrait of the collaborative process as inclusive. It introduces recommendations for local health care reform by first describing the way the recommendations were reached: as the product of "the consensus development process." Consensus-building represents a format commonly used for negotiation among U.N. and development organizations that strives to include representatives of all relevant social groups in negotiation and policy formation. The report describes a negotiation process in which conference participants were divided into topical discussion groups led by one representative from St. Petersburg and one international advisor and undertook "several hours of vigorous discussion and debate." Without providing insights into specifics areas of disagreement or concern, the report then asserts that the groups concluded by reaching consensus: "At the end of the meeting, it was clear that the final recommendations were made both by and for the people of St. Petersburg" (WHO 1993a: 5).

This portrait of unanimity is followed by over five pages of recommendations for Russian maternity care, covering services around prenatal care, birth, the postpartum period, neonatal care, and family planning. It advises that maternity services be reformed to establish "continuity of care throughout pregnancy and labor, based on one-to-one care." Recommendations for changing health care practices during birth assert that "the environment of the maternity hospital should be friendlier to the women receiving care . . . women should give birth in separate rooms with all due privacy; women should be able to make choices about their labor and delivery (on such issues as their mobility and position); partners and other chosen visitors should have access to mothers and their babies throughout their stay in the maternity hospital" (1993a: 6). Postpartum reforms included the need for maternity hospitals to "practice rooming-in, allowing babies to remain with their mothers 24 hours a day" and a recommendation for city administrators "to finance free contraceptives for women after they give birth" (1993a: 7). Neonatal care was to focus on the encouragement of breastfeeding (1993a: 8). Throughout all spheres of maternal and reproductive health, including family planning services, explicit recommendations were made for the development of local self-help and community support groups (1993a: 10). This list of "possible solutions" for improving maternal health also included the following statement: "In a free society, women make informed choices about their health care, and health professionals serve rather than dominate their patients" (1993a: 4).

With this programmatic assertion, the claim that a consensus emerged among conference participants is rendered somewhat dubious. One wonders why continued training projects would be perceived as necessary if Russian providers really accepted these principles. Moreover, because the report does not attribute any statements to particular individuals or groups, we have little insight into who among conference participants enthusiastically embraced this view and who may have expressed (or silently held) doubts. The report fails to discuss how the "vigorous debates" were transformed into unanimous agreements in reaching recommendations for reform. Indeed, the image of consensus is possible only because the participants at the conference are presented as a homogeneous mass, speaking in a singular voice, with unanimity and agreement their predetermined, and ultimately realized, goal.

Without doubt, the recommended reforms, such as giving women choice about their medical care and ensuring them full access to their babies and relatives in the hospital, held the promise of significantly increasing women's sense of control and feelings of safety in birth. At the same time, this report begs the question about the kinds of methods global experts deployed to promote such reforms, methods that would have both ethical and pragmatic implications. The report's emphasis on "consensus building" serves rhetorically to acknowledge that the character of global interventions is an ethical issue. Like the concept of "community participation" (Morgan 1993), the "consensus" strategy expresses development institutions' intention to construct assistance as a fundamentally inclusive and noncoercive, democratic project. Yet without details about competing views and interests, the depiction of the recommendations as the products of unqualified agreement had the effect of sidelining questions about power relations between the global advisors and the Russian participants. Reaching consensus may actually have ended up silencing minority perspectives or unpopular opinions, rather than delving into their logics and rationales. Ironically, such pragmatic use of discourse to signify the development team's compliance with accepted norms of international assistance bears an uncanny resemblance to the use of language by Soviet Party officials before Perestroika (Yurchak 2003).

DEMOCRACY RHETORIC IN A
DEVELOPMENT FRAMEWORK

My doubts that a genuine consensus was reached in 1992 were substantiated when I saw later developments in the WHO–St. Petersburg collaboration. By summer 1994, when I began a period of long-term fieldwork examining the WHO–St. Petersburg project, city officials demonstrated overt apathy toward the project. I arrived expecting to document two years' worth of local improvisations with Healthy Cities Project ideals, but found instead that the St. Petersburg project office had done nothing in terms of coordinating, developing, or expanding the project. WHO literature in Russian lay untouched on the bookshelves in the Healthy Cities Project office, collecting dust. Institutions designated model WHO projects worked in isolation from each other and from the Healthy Cities Project office. The office boasting a "WHO—Healthy Cities Project" sign on its door had forged no ties with local women's NGOs and had shown virtually no interest in promoting multi-sectoral links or community outreach. Office staff were busy engaging some of the other global collaborators that beckoned; they devoted their time to cultivating relations with global pharmaceutical companies, documentary film crews, and other foreigners eager to pay for their services. In face-to-face meetings with visiting WHO consultants, members of the Public Health Committee affirmed their commitment to the project and emphasized the achievements their work in maternal health had brought. Yet, as one European-based Healthy Cities Project official noted privately with incomprehension and resentment, St. Petersburg's Public Health Committee repeatedly neglected to mention the maternal health projects associated with WHO in their publications on health-care reform. (Instead of pursuing WHO-inspired concerns, local planners were consumed with the reorganization of health care financing, transferring financial responsibility for health care away from the state to insurance companies and enterprises.) Frustration on the part of WHO officials was growing, while Russian public health experts were too consumed by other matters to give their relations with the Healthy Cities Project much thought. In December 1994 a secretary in the St. Petersburg Healthy Cities Project office explained the local attitude toward WHO's programs to me in blunt terms: "Look, a job as a bureaucrat for the [St. Petersburg] Public Health Committee doesn't pay anything. WHO doesn't fund this office either. You can't expect people to work for free. . . . [Global] pharmaceutical companies . . . are [the ones] paying us. They are determining priorities for the city's health policy now."

This secretary's dismissive stance toward WHO was echoed multiple times by her boss, St. Petersburg's representative to WHO. This official, hired by the city's Public Health Committee to head the St. Petersburg Healthy Cities Project Office, frequently accused the international agency of completely neglecting St. Petersburg's needs. "WHO has done nothing for the city. We need money!" she would insist bluntly, revealing her complete disregard of the global organization's official role in the project and her city's own written commitments to invest economically in the population's needs.

The principles of the Healthy Cities Project—that municipal government would dedicate substantial resources to achieving WHO's visions of equity and a social model of health and would make concerted efforts to promote multi-sectoral action for health reforms—had not been fulfilled by St. Petersburg. As I visited the three state health care institutions that had been identified with the Healthy Cities Project, I saw that they had significantly transformed their approach to reproductive health care, in ways that sometimes coincided with and sometimes contravened WHO's recommendations. They were promoting breastfeeding, family planning, and a reduction in the number of abortions. Some were undertaking education for health providers and lay persons in the form of community outreach (Rivkin-Fish 1999). On the other hand, as I discuss in Chapter 2, principles of women's autonomy and equity in health care had been neither accepted nor incorporated in these or other state health care institutions. The maternity hospital had instituted mother-baby rooming-in and experimented with visiting hours and allowing companions during labor for all patients. Still, providers explained that procedures such as enemas, episiotomies, and shaving remained routine and compulsory. They had not adopted the idea that women needed to have a degree of autonomy in their birth experiences, but explained how they appreciated rooming-in for lightening their own work loads. And while the procedures of mother-baby rooming-in and companions during labor had spread beyond the model site to other city hospitals, as WHO envisioned, most had done so not according to the agency's principles that companions entailed women's "basic right in birth," but as a luxury service available only to those patients willing and able to pay.

Soon after beginning fieldwork, I realized that the method of promoting change by offering a blueprint for action, a set of guidelines for being accepted into the club of Healthy Cities, did not lead to ideological change. The city invested the minimal amount of resources necessary to gain membership without ceding political power to community groups or creating a more pluralistic framework for public health debate and dialogue. Despite the impasse with the local Healthy Cities officials, WHO did not review or reconsider its cooperation with the city. In private conversations about the project, agency officials attributed the successes and limitations of the project to individual personalities in the Public Health Committee. They did not seek to understand the roles of global and local political-economic forces, from the World Bank and IMF to St. Petersburg's policymakers—with their productive relations with global pharmaceutical firms—or the city's indifference to the Healthy Cities Project. In fact, as these forces actively aimed to minimize public responsibility for welfare provision and enable the semi-privatization of services, they indirectly contributed to the stunted development of the Healthy Cities Project's outcomes.

Notwithstanding the tepid interest that local officials showed in WHO's calls for equity and women's rights, the consultants continued to pursue their agendas in the city. In late 1994, a Healthy Cities Project official from Copenhagen arrived in St. Petersburg to announce that an independent team of maternal health experts affiliated with WHO had secured bilateral funding for a two-year series of professional training workshops for Russian maternal health providers. Workshops would examine topics such as the appropriate use of technology in birth and the importance of focusing on individual empowerment and social well-being for improving women's health. Their grant applications and project descriptions emphasized the success of programs already undertaken, such as the establishment of the Healthy Cities Project and its model institutions.

EDUCATION FOR DEMOCRACY

From the point of view of development agencies, training workshops for health providers represented an exemplary method of intervention. Because it transfers expertise rather than material resources, educational programming has been viewed as an ideal way to minimize the potential for assistance to be extorted and misappropriated (Bivens in Abramson 1999). Yet development projects have not systematically considered the appropriateness of education programming as a method for inducing specific forms of change in local public health practices. For example, the question of whether recipients targeted for aid perceive a need for retraining is not typically a condition for project funding. Indeed, because development projects in former Soviet states have worked with the assumption that Western models represented both technical superiority and ideological victory over state socialism (Cohen 2000), Western experts were presumed competent to judge what kinds of knowledge and skills local experts lacked (Rivkin-Fish 2004b; Wedel 2001). When I introduced my goals of studying Russian's perspectives on maternal health reform to the consultants, I found that only one delegation member had considered the feasibility of inspiring a concern with women's self-determination by teaching Russian health care providers about it. This consultant had a graduate degree in education and conducted outreach on contraceptives for a pharmaceutical firm.

I conducted intensive participant-observation during WHO's training workshops. Consultants' presentations covered topics ranging from the causes of maternal morbidity and mortality to the importance of evidence-based medical practice, breastfeeding, reduction of unnecessary interventions during birth, and women's having choices about their care. I listened to the formal comments and informal asides each group made and noted examples of how the skillful simultaneous translator sometimes adapted or altered meanings in the effort to keep up with the lively pace of interaction. I focus here on the tactics by which consultants tried to catalyze change in participants' approach to women's care, the rhetorical modes of persuasion consultants deployed to "train" local providers. Their arguments expressed their own culturally rooted assumptions about Russian political change, professional power, and gender identity, assumptions that did not ring true to Russians' experiences. Moreover, while consultants' rhetoric rendered certain dimensions of provider-patient interactions visible and made them the object of critical discourse, they simultaneously overlooked the inequalities shaping these relations, such as the institutional foundations of provider-patient conflicts and physicians' constrained forms of social authority. In response, Russian health providers

deflected WHO's analyses and denied both the value and practical relevance of autonomy for women as a component of health reform. As we
will see below, as providers drew on their everyday experiences in the clinic
to justify their practices and pose alternative health reform priorities, they
partially exposed how the configuration of structural inequalities shaping
women's health care in Russia differed from what WHO assumed it to be.
Finally, the workshop debates and interviews with delegates reveal how
WHO made sense of Russian providers' perceptions through their *own*
framework of assumptions. When faced with issues that did not fit into
their preconceived agenda of reform, consultants were left to devise arguments through on-the-spot improvisations. Their responses played out the
structured limitations of the development paradigm by shifting attention
away from the political and economic factors that Russian participants
discussed. In this way, consultants inadvertently demonstrated how thoroughly they had internalized the structural possibilities and limitations of
promoting democracy within the development framework.

THE WHO–ST. PETERSBURG MATERNAL
MORTALITY WORKSHOP

It was a snowy week in March 1995 when approximately thirty-five of
St. Petersburg's maternal health planners, physicians, midwives, and nurses
gathered in the conference room of one maternity hospital located in the
south of the city. The WHO delegation conducted the same workshop
twice in the course of a week, repeating it in order to be able to include
several representatives from each of the city's eleven maternity hospitals
while keeping the groups small enough to permit discussions. The workshop agenda comprised three full working days of lectures, discussions,
slides, and role-playing intended to introduce Russian health providers to
the ways birth and the postnatal period are cared for in the West and to
promote the adoption of recommended reforms in St. Petersburg. Consultants agreed to my requests to participate in and observe these workshops and to interview them as part of my study of the cultural dimensions of development work. The only condition they placed on my study
was that I was to keep certain identifying aspects of their project confidential, a protocol that fit completely within anthropological ethical standards for protecting informants.[7] While personally open and eager to discuss their work with me (and thus gracious in allowing me to conduct this
study), consultants were conceptually unprepared to address the anthropological kinds of concerns I would be raising.

The delegation was led by Kathy Nelson, a psychologist and specialist
in childbirth education; Dr. Kevin Daniels, an obstetrician and pediatri-

cian who was a long-time activist in the Western movement to reform childbirth procedures; Dr. William Warren, an obstetrician who has been involved in reforming medical school curricula to emphasize nonhierarchical modes of teaching and practicing medicine; Susan Jones, a midwifery activist; Andrea Smith, a nurse who specialized in neonatal care; and Arthur Henderson, the educational representative from a North American pharmaceutical firm. Standing at the front of the conference room, the delegates constructed their arguments and presented their data with the aid of an overhead projector, a VCR, photocopied handouts, and the help of a Russian interpreter who translated simultaneously between English and Russian. Sitting together in the audience were the senior maternal health policymakers of the St. Petersburg Public Health Committee, head doctors from several city maternity hospitals, and physicians, midwives, and nurses whose daily professional activity was limited to the clinic setting. The delegates focused the workshop on the care of women during and after birth, alternatively presenting descriptions of hospital birth and home birth in the West and articulating explicit suggestions for reforms in St. Petersburg. Common to virtually all workshop presentations was the delegates' conviction that the problem of maternal mortality could be largely addressed through reforming the provider-patient relationship. Drawing on the Canadian National Guidelines for maternity care, they presented concrete suggestions for clinical reforms within a broader ideology of obstetrics care known as "family-centered maternity care." This model of obstetrics envisions a demedicalized health care setting in which the needs of women and their families become the priorities of health providers. In the afternoon of the first day of the workshop, Kathy Nelson outlined the basic principles of the philosophy that would frame future discussions of all recommended clinical reforms:

1. Care is oriented to the woman's individual need.
2. Birth is a healthy event, unique for each woman.
3. The woman has autonomy in decision-making.
4. Women choose their health care professionals to assist, not direct, them.
5. Relationships between women, families, and health providers are based on mutual respect and trust.
6. Women and their families have full knowledge about their care and the circumstances surrounding it.

Copies of these principles, in Russian, were handed out to all participants for future reference, for these were the building blocks of all recommended reforms. Nonetheless, WHO consultants took pains not to appear as if they were imposing their approach on local practitioners. Representing the principles as "recommended guidelines, not rules," they simultaneously strove to acknowledge that conditions differ among countries, while still asserting that the basic principles underlying this model of care were universally appropriate. Summarizing the six guiding principles, Bill Warren self-consciously tried to maintain this delicate balance: "It's different to implement change in St. Petersburg and [a North American city]; all areas have their particularities with family-centered maternity care. We're talking about giving more power to families and less power to institutions." Nonetheless, neither he nor other WHO consultants ever gave examples of what they considered such differences might be or invited further discussion on this topic.

The workshop's sessions proceeded to examine specific clinical problems through the lens of family-centered maternity care principles. Consultants justified all recommendations by repeatedly asserting that pregnancy is a normal, healthy experience and need not be automatically targeted for biomedical interventions. Several discussions were devoted to the "appropriate use of technology" in pregnancy and the use of routine procedures surrounding labor and delivery. Consultants explained that their concerns with these issues centered on two overriding themes: the scientific effectiveness of medical interventions and the psychological effect of such interventions on women's experiences of pregnancy and childbirth. Asserting that recent research in the U.S. proved that the routine use of ultrasound was found to have no impact on fetal outcome, they characterized its widespread routinization as a prime example of the undue medicalization of pregnancy. Rather then employing specific technologies according to their proven medical benefits, consultants argued, physicians are often swayed by society's fascination with technology. "I have a favorite saying that explains this love of technology," added Kevin Daniels, in an unmistakably critical tone: "The difference between men and boys is the price of their toys!"

In a related discussion, consultants referred to more studies in North America that provided support for demedicalizing women's care during birth. In particular, they noted that common pre-labor procedures such as shaving the pubic area and administering enemas do not contribute to decreased infection rates, as had been previously assumed. Rather, these are medically insignificant interventions, and should be entirely discontinued. WHO consultants emphasized that shaving women and giving them enemas create a mechanical approach to birth that undermines women's comfort and control over their bodies. When one Russian health provider loudly retorted that "women would surely rather have enemas than defecate during labor," WHO consultants argued that women should at least be given the chance to decide for themselves whether they want the procedure or not. In a similar vein, consultants argued that the episiotomy rate should be reduced.[8] Characterizing it as yet another routine procedure that contributes to the medicalized character of birth, they explained that research has demonstrated that episiotomies cause increased pain and discomfort for women and may actually increase, rather than reduce, the risk of tearing. Providers could minimize the use of episiotomy by caring for each woman as an individual, devoting time to her needs, and not automatically assuming the need for a medical intervention, Susan explained. This argument drew on the experiences of midwives in the West who devote intensive efforts to massaging the perineum to avoid tears or minimize their severity. Susan encouraged Russian colleagues to reconsider their roles in serving women, explaining, "It requires caregivers to take the time and be patient and work with the woman to avoid the episiotomy."

As an important aspect of promoting women's comfort and autonomous decision-making during birth, consultants advocated that the family be at the center of the pregnancy and birth experience. During the first afternoon of the workshop, they showed a video to illustrate "what family-centered care looks like in clinical practice—what it means when we as midwives, nurses, and doctors directly work with families." The video presented husbands and older siblings attending prenatal care visits with the expectant mother, health providers sitting and enthusiastically answering the family's questions, and entire families eagerly supporting the laboring mother during the birth itself. Consultants emphasized that fathers' and children's involvement in a woman's pregnancy is very important, and requires health providers to be flexible when working with patients. Again, they stressed the need to make birth "a personal experience." "The most important thing," Susan added as she shut off the VCR and turned toward the participants, "is to focus on individual needs." In presenting these portraits of family-centered birth, consultants applauded the video-filmed caregivers for providing personal attention and customized care to each individual woman and family.

RUSSIAN HEALTH PROVIDERS RESPOND

Both overtly and covertly, Russian health providers rejected the arguments WHO presented during the workshop. Senior officials in the Public Health Committee and chief doctors of maternity homes were the only participants to object directly to the foreign delegation; physicians, midwives, and nurses deferred to the political elites in their midst and refrained from making their opinions public during the workshop. Those who did express dissent struggled to refute WHO's assumptions that Russian women's pregnancies were healthy and that prioritizing the fulfillment of individual needs and choice would positively affect health outcomes. One telling moment came at the end of the first day of the workshop, when the head of the WHO delegation, Kathy Nelson, asked the participants which aspects of the proposed reforms they were in favor of implementing. After an awkward silence, one of the city's leading maternal health administrators rose to answer the question. At first measured, her speech quickly transformed into a passionate outburst as she enumerated the litany of problems that confront health providers on a daily basis:

> We have extremely high numbers of risk groups, the structure of sickness, a high rate of neonatal infections due to intrauterine infections, 80 percent have bacterial vaginitis, and this leads to low immunity, and also extra-genital problems, eclampsia, all different problems, scars on the uterus, chlamydia, yeast infections. There are many problems and they are all together, in combination. We therefore have no women who could go without these [technologies and routine] treatments. . . . Syphilis and gonorrhea have recently increased twenty times. We know it's related to our poverty, the poverty of our government. We're beginning to be affectionate [*laskovyi*] to women, we can let a woman have her husband come in [during the birth], but we can't change everything only by being nice.

Through this cascade of pathologies, she identified a range of obstacles not acknowledged by WHO experts and instantly discounted their recommendations that technologies and routine procedures be reduced. Up until that point, WHO's insistence that Russian health providers minimize the importance of technology in childbirth stemmed from the recognition that improvements in social and environmental conditions play a far greater role in raising the overall levels of public health than does the isolated accumulation of medical techniques and machines. With this comment, the city official in maternal health redirected the issue at stake, defining the urgent problem for health providers as being *how to deal with* the health consequences of poor and worsening socioeconomic conditions. Caricaturing WHO's agenda as insignificant with her statement "We can't change everything only by being nice," she argued that in the absence of significant political and financial investment in health amidst conditions of spiraling morbidity, a reliance on technology was the only feasible way of ensuring the minimum medical capacity to cope with dire health problems. In the eyes of WHO consultants, these objections only served to confirm their suspicions that Russian experts stubbornly clung to a model that prized technology, medical expertise, and the need for medical dominance over women.

RHETORICS OF PERSUASION I: MAKE USE OF YOUR DEMOCRATIC FREEDOMS

This debate over the use of technology encapsulated the diverging agendas of Russians and the WHO. Russian health providers had come to discuss clinical techniques, a topic they considered appropriate to their standing as medical experts. WHO sought to persuade health providers that the use of technology was part of the problem, not the solution, and that improving women's health required providers to cede authority over care in birth to their patients. On the first day of the workshop, Kathy Nelson tried to link the promotion of women's rights in health with the more general political autonomy that the Russian city had expressed in their collaboration with WHO. Her comments aroused one of the most candid debates of either workshop, in which St. Petersburg health providers challenged not only the existence of a "consensus" on the kinds of reforms needed, but policymakers' sincere commitment to the Healthy Cities maternal health project. In portraying the city's political agreement as empty rhetoric alone, health providers led WHO in a meta-discussion on the sources and agents of social change. Nelson began by asserting, "We think it's important that you begin to ask women what they want, what they like, and don't like, and that you take it into account in giving care. Everything we do is based on specific principles. The first is self-determination: When we began three years ago, the city of St. Petersburg decided itself that maternal and child health is a priority."

The chief doctor of one city maternity home, a burly man with an aggressive tone, interrupted the WHO leader and provocatively inquired: "What do you mean by 'priority'?"

Kevin Daniels interjected: "The biggest problem of health in St. Petersburg is maternal and child health."

The chief doctor did not accept this as an answer, and challenged the WHO to discuss the practical outcomes of the above-mentioned "decision": "At the Consensus conference did you hear an affirmation of priorities from the mayor, including a financial commitment? Because WE haven't heard it."

Daniels attempted to address the doctors' frustrations by emphasizing the constancy of the WHO's democratic approach:

> The politicians in the mayor's office said, "We need this program and we want it." I know it's frustrating for people who work in clinics that politicians aren't giving enough. . . . Our seminar is founded on the principle of democracy. Those who attended the 1992 conference know that we tried to include everyone in decisions about recommendations through democratic ways. . . . And the care for women and children should also be democratic; people who get services should have the right to say what they feel about the kind of care they get. It's what we call self-determination when the people themselves decide what they want to do and fix, so it's not people from the outside coming to tell you what's wrong with you. We also have a democratic approach. In Western Europe and in other systems it's changing. Before

it was doctors and professors who decided what all other professionals should do. Now it's all the people together, including patients, who, together with doctors, decide. So democracy is coming to medical institutions, hospitals, and clinics.

Clearly exasperated, a second male chief doctor (the only other man among the Russian participants) interjected and argued that local conditions, from women's low awareness to political intransigence, were barriers to implementing WHO's project:

> The first problem is that in [your country] women think of their health differently than how our women here do. Here it's the last thing that women care about. That's why it's often not a medical problem but a political-economic and social problem. Thanks to your program we see how people in England and Finland care about their health. But here it's the last priority. And it's not our public health policy to prioritize this among our population. . . . We're dealing with more than seventy years of history in which health was [addressed] only with words. Financially, health received the last priority even then, and now we see no changes in the politics.

Kathy Nelson countered by turning the discussion away from city public health politics to reiterate the notion of individual empowerment and self-determination for health providers themselves, "You are the people who can change what you do everyday. You can't change the government, but you can change what you do. We're bringing you information and it's up to you to decide what you want to do and what's not relevant for you."

This exchange exemplified the communicative performances that both sides staged throughout the three-day workshops. Russian health providers challenged the consultants' assertion that the city was committed to improving maternal health, and they dissociated themselves from the apparently duplicitous politicians who signed the reform agreement. They contested WHO's implication that the agreement itself, made in the name of "the city of St. Petersburg," proved that local self-determination was at work in public health policymaking. Rather than seeing the agreement as a sign of actual financial and political commitment, they countered that their experiences over the last three years led them to discount the city's official statements as merely evidence of the continued hypocrisy of politicians. Claiming that "We're dealing with more than seventy years of history in which health was only in words . . . and now we see no changes in politics," health providers did more than dismiss the city's agreement with WHO as yet another example of meaningless political propaganda. Implicitly, they also revealed their own sense of being disempowered, as alienated from the policymaking process now as they had been prior to democratic reforms. Workshop participants perceived WHO experts, by shifting the discussion away from city public health politics to providers' ability to "change what you do everyday," to be dismissing the very relevance of a political-level commitment for improving women's health.

WHO representatives might have confronted Russians' objections with questions to help clarify the kinds of dilemmas Russians faced in women's health. The opportunity for a dialogue existed, for the global officials actually had some first-hand experience with the St. Petersburg government's duplicity, as they observed its neglect for the Healthy Cities Project. Just prior to the workshop, the St. Petersburg Committee of Public Health had made *no mention* of the maternal health project or women's health in general in its most recent publication. The entire booklet was devoted to celebrating the new system of medical insurance and budgetary accounting (Public Health Committee 1994). (City officials forwarded an English-language version of the document to WHO officials, leaving Copenhagen experts bristling at the glaring omission.) Some of the workshop leaders knew of this slight. Yet they avoided discussing the city's policies in the public context of the workshop. They neither pursued the question of whether St. Petersburg politicians really were committed to improving women's reproductive health, investigated whether Russian health providers had political influence on public health policies, nor inquired into the financial straits plaguing city health institutions. Missing this opportunity, they failed to acknowledge the particular disadvantages health providers who worked in the clinic faced as they attempted to cope with problems their policymakers ignored.

Instead, consultants steered the discussion away from their audience's concerns. In striving rhetorically to salvage the concept of self-determination, they insisted that democratic reforms must develop through individual initiative and not only through the agency of state politics. Minimizing the failures of local politicians to act in good faith, and not considering the increasing hegemony of neoliberal policies, they didactically instructed health providers that despite the lack of funding and perceived political stagnation, each one of them, as individuals, was still capable of introducing reforms "in what you do everyday."

I sat in these lectures achingly torn between my convictions as a feminist and my anthropological commitment to listen and understand these contrasting ethical positions. Feeling caught between two moral worlds, I did not publicly speak during the workshops themselves. I worked intensely during breaks, at lunches, and on the subway ride home each day to gather Russian participants' views and reactions. I set up interviews to hear their perspectives in greater depth in the weeks following the workshops. I strove to understand the different conditions and experiences that generated the contrasting ethical positions. I tried to intervene behind the scenes with WHO consultants, to highlight the constraints Russians were facing and provoke discussion of how these differences might be addressed. One consultant, annoyed with my insistent questions about how he understood the project and its methods, suggested sarcastically that I could call his work "imperialism" in the name of women's rights. I did not consider the term "imperialism" an accurate description of this project. But the word did highlight my concerns with power and difference in the global interaction in a way no other term I could think of did.

RHETORICS OF PERSUASION II: "RECOGNIZE YOUR OWN INTERESTS AS WOMEN"

Because WHO Healthy Cities Project officials were unwilling or unable to pressure politicians about their policies on women's health, the delegation had only rhetorical means to try to gain health providers' sympathy to the cause of women's autonomy in the clinic. Workshop consultants could have acknowledged to the Russians that their political-economic problems were real and/or raised the importance of these issues to WHO officials with the Healthy Cities Project. But having identified so closely with the limited parameters of action established by the development paradigm, they never considered doing so. At the end of the first, long day of the workshop filled with back-to-back discussions, presentations, and debates, Kathy Nelson turned to the thirty or so women obstetricians, midwives, and nurses sitting before her and attempted to change the tone of the discussion. Noting that her audience included merely two men, Nelson addressed her Russian colleagues with an emotional plea to remember their own experiences in childbirth, asserting:

> If I can ask you who had children to remember your own feelings, having your feet up in stirrups, uncovered, with the door open, people walking around and you've been shaved and had your bowels cleaned out, and there's nobody around you who you love and trust. Women became very uncomfortable with this in our part of the world, and wanted it no more. And women were happy to learn that the research supports them. Women want to enjoy the process of having a baby. They want to feel safe and loved and they want dignity and privacy in this experience.

Informing this rhetorical strategy was Nelson's assumption that the importance doctors placed on their professional identities would naturally be surpassed by their identification with other women, *even in the context of professional work.* Russian health providers, however, rejected this appeal, as one workshop participant sitting near me muttered to her colleagues, "Our women are used to being told what to do." Indeed, throughout the workshop Russian participants' comments revealed how they separated themselves as experts from the population at large and constructed patients as a distinct social category—as "our women" [*nashi zhenshchiny*] or "patients" [*bol'nye*]. It was precisely through their images of women as other—as ill and incapable of dealing with autonomy in decision-making—that women health providers constructed their own identities—as authoritative professionals. This distinction emerged most insistently in response to WHO's claim that demedicalizing the health sphere would improve maternal health. Russian health providers deemed WHO's assertions that "pregnancy is a normal, healthy condition" to be true "abroad," "for their women," but certainly not a valid description of the reproductive experiences of "our women." As the maternal health planner cited above, Russians portrayed almost all of their patients as suffering from serious complications throughout their pregnancies and in need of close medical surveillance. Valia, an obstetrician who participated in the workshop, unambiguously rejected the idea of relinquishing authority to promote patients' independence or responsibility: "If I ask a woman if she *wants* an enema, she'll say, I don't [even] want to push. . . . If a woman comes to me and says 'I want a healthy baby,' then she has to listen to the doctor."

In attempting to promote Russian women's autonomy and equality through the re-education of health providers, consultants could only devise appeals based on cultural assumptions and ad-hoc psychological presumptions about what would persuade doctors to change their attitudes. The appeal to women doctors "to remember your own experiences in birth" seemed, to consultants coming from the male-dominated medical profession in the West, a promising tactic. For Russian women health providers, it was not.

"EMPOWERMENT" WITHIN A DEVELOPMENT MODEL

At some levels, the delegates themselves were aware that their project entailed both subtle and overt forms of power. Yet as we saw in the report on the Consensus Conference, this awareness emerged through formulaic kinds of acknowledgments, such as when consultants self-consciously sought to portray the conference's recommendations as an outcome based in global-local "consensus," without giving any details of how conflicts and difference were negotiated and overcome. When interviewed about how they dealt with differences in cultural knowledge (which is related to their deployment of power), consultants responded in similarly equivocal ways. They were at once keenly conscious of women patients' disempowerment in health care and strikingly unaware of how their own intervention sidelined broader political questions, both about global and state policies and about their actual methods of inducing change. Daniels described the delegation's work as bringing change, in a unidirectional way, to Russia. He spoke of ideas as things brought to Russians, not the mutual outcomes of relationships: "This is the first step in a thousand-mile trek; it'll take decades if not generations, if ever. If this country does incorporate the spirit of democracy and not autocracy, they'll do it one individual at a time. If you get one person out of a thousand to rethink, you're an enormous success. We throw out a lot of ideas and hope some of them will be picked up."

The metaphor of "throwing out ideas" and having them "picked up" was echoed in interviews I conducted with other delegates, who, in attempts at modesty, described their goals in Russia as "planting the seeds" of democratic ideas. Though undoubtedly sincere, this appeal to modesty had important effects—it construed "ideas" as akin to commodities— seemingly available for any individual to choose according to her desire and whim—and unattached to the structural positions and interests of those who espouse them. With this discourse, consultants established a project of promoting women's empowerment by educating doctors about "the idea" of offering women patients rights, even if politicians lied and failed to fulfill their economic commitments and no legislative or political guarantees of women's rights were in place. By isolating "ideas" from the broader structural processes they are embedded in, and not simultaneously insisting on changes in those structures and political processes, consultants could blame Russian doctors and policymakers who did not "pick up" the ideas of women's rights and social well-being, as being blind, obstinate, and hungry for power.

The view that "democracy" could emerge in women's health care through will power alone, as "one person at a time" accepted the "spirit" of this new idea, was further expressed by the delegation's leader. I asked Kathy Nelson to explain her rhetorical strategies, and specifically, why she decided to appeal to Russian health providers' own experiences in childbirth. As we sat together in the bar of her St. Petersburg hotel, she shared her understanding of how the "dehumanized" quality of maternal health care reflected the ubiquitous dehumanization of all social relationships in Soviet society. The dilemma, she claimed, had to do with the suppression of emotion, a problem that Westerners could effectively help Russians to transcend:

> Their ballet expresses such phenomenal warmth and feeling. . . . It's there in the culture, it's just not been allowed to express itself in the work world, in the medical world. That was stamped out under the old system. . . . It was a very mechanical,

mechanistic process of birth, and the emotive side of birth was not allowed to express itself. Just as it was between people, people would also not be allowed to trust
each other, share thoughts, feelings, hopes. If you said the wrong thing, you were
punished. Or betrayed . . . But I don't believe [humanism's] not there. It's deeply
ingrained in the tradition. You see it in the art and music and ballet. All that we are
doing is awakening that and giving permission to have it again.

Similar to Daniels's comments above, this explanation functioned to
bypass questions and answers about the need for political-economic kinds
of changes to ensure women's empowerment in health care. Nelson viewed
the problems women patients experienced at the hands of their health
providers as resolvable by submitting doctors to a kind of social-psycho-
logical therapy. The problem with this view, of course, is that the image of
Russian work settings beset by the terror of totalitarian repression and
betrayal, with colleagues utterly estranged from one another, was founded
on Cold War fantasies about Russia, rather than any genuine understanding of local workplace dynamics. As we will see, providers and patients
experienced a variety of kinds of relations and interactions, including intensely intimate bonds of friendship. Hospital staff members enjoyed
strong camaraderie as well, if within lines of vertical hierarchical difference. And to the extent that any relations of hierarchy and power were
locally perceived to be problematic, the notion that they would be overcome once Westerners "gave permission" for Russians to change belied a
hubris of extraordinary proportions.

Working according to the assumptions embedded in governmentality
led consultants to hold several depoliticized visions of what their intervention was doing—from "forming consensus" to "throwing out ideas" to
"giving permission" for the expression of emotions. Without intentionally
denying politics, consultants' use of these images as they conceptualized
their own tasks had the inadvertent affect of cutting off questions related
to larger political processes, such as how providers' domination over patients might be related to physician deprofessionalization, patient disenfranchisement, and the increasing poverty of both groups amidst market
reforms. These images also deflected attention away from the question of
how their own intervention involved the deployment of power.

Despite its rhetoric of promoting women's rights, this project was unable to address the fact that empowering women in health care required
extensive changes in political-economic policies. Instead, their struggle for
"women's rights" became an ideological campaign alone, one that could
not acknowledge that women and providers need practical resources to
demand new legal guarantees and ensure their enforcement. In this way,
the concomitant work by state authorities and global forces to constrain

health care provisions and create the conditions whereby women were impoverished and therefore at constant risk for disease was conceptually pushed aside. The possibility that certain structural conditions prevented women doctors and patients from viewing themselves in alignment with each other and accepting the notion of patient empowerment remained unexplored.

WORKSHOP RESULTS

Inadvertently, the limits of this project design gave rise to several unintended consequences, another systemic feature of development interventions (Ferguson 1994; Lemke 2000). The most immediate effect of this workshop was that Russian health providers recognized that the concepts of democracy and women's rights were being deployed in rhetorical ways, and they found WHO's arguments trivial. Inasmuch as the concrete reforms recommended in the name of "democracy" seemed disassociated from health providers' practical experiences and daily problems in the clinic, the value of "women's rights" appeared negligible. In conversations I had with Russian participants during lunches, coffee breaks, and in the weeks following the workshop, their criticisms targeted precisely the decontextualized character of WHO's recommendations for health care reform. Russian health providers repeatedly told me that the recommendations were irrelevant for the local context, because they took into account neither the realities of Russian life nor the crises of Russian health care. One obstetrician who participated in the workshop, Anna Valerievna, explained: "In the past, midwives came here and worked with us clinically. Midwives came here not to check on our work but to work together. This was good. They could see and understand our conditions. If these [WHO representatives] would experience working in these conditions for themselves, then they could suggest something concrete for us."

When I asked Anna Valerievna how she evaluated WHO's recommendations, she did not mention the issues of democracy or women's self-determination; her response implicitly characterized these notions as disconnected from the daily problems facing health providers and women who need health care. The obstetrician quoted earlier, Valia, was incensed over the delegates' "meaningless" approach for Russia's problems. Craving an exchange of medical knowledge and the opportunity to discuss clinical problems, she instead described encountering didactic, moral "models of behavior." Fuming, she asserted:

> We wanted them to give us information about medical procedures. They won't get socialism out of us, but they could teach us about their concrete practices. We don't

need to be given models about how to behave with one another, we have an information famine. We want them to tell us the concrete details about how they work in specific circumstances. . . . [For example] Do you do c-sections by yourself or with partners?[9]

Secondly, Valia resented that the structure of the workshop entailed training sessions in which "they talked and we listened." Valia portrayed the workshop in vividly colonialist (and racist) symbolism:

> The delegates' attitude toward us was of missionaries who came to teach the monkeys [sic]. We're good specialists and have a lot of experience. Doctors at this workshop had as much as eighteen years experience in maternity hospitals. . . . We could teach them a lot. If we could've talked about organizational issues, we could also help them with examples of pathological births, criminal abortions, and situations of women in poverty. We can help you learn how to do these things, but nobody wanted to hear it.

When I asked Valia how she would have liked WHO to organize the workshop, her answer provided telling insights into her desire for experiencing professional equality in exchanges with foreign delegations: "Come on, Michele, how do you organize an international conference? A committee decides in advance what's important. Send us abstracts about what you want to discuss ahead of time, and we'll decide if we need it or not. We respect our own time and yours. So send us your ideas in advance and we won't sit here for three days angry and frustrated."

Valia was incensed that her professional knowledge was not acknowledged as equal to Western medical standards. She proposed an alternative genre of exchange centering on dialogue—a research conference—where decision-making power about priorities for discussion would be distributed among Russians and international consultants as peers. Although I found many of Valia's images of provider power and women's subordination disturbing, I had to agree that her image of an international exchange of ideas and dialogue seemed a more "democratic" model of interactions than either "consensus" or "training."

EPILOGUE

Sitting in that hospital auditorium during those heady March days in 1995, I experienced an unnerving mix of emotions as WHO urged Russian obstetricians to respect women's needs in birth. Consultants' arguments spoke directly to my own concerns that the values of individual autonomy and women's self-determination must be paramount to the organization of reproductive services. I wholeheartedly agreed that pregnancy and birth were healthy processes, and their medicalization around the world reflected political and cultural forms of domination, rather than beneficial technological advancements that improved birth outcomes. Four years later, I would draw on the same critiques when I sought out care for my own pregnancy and birth in the U.S.

The overwhelmingly negative responses that Russian providers expressed to these claims disturbed me, but also begged for analysis. How was it that women obstetricians and midwives, almost all of whom had given birth themselves, refused to acknowledge the systemic experiences of humiliation, vulnerability, and subordination that women patients appeared to face when institutions afforded them so little control over their bodies and births? My anthropological training left me unsatisfied with the answers provided by one WHO consultant, that "doctors everywhere want to keep power for themselves." And my personal experiences with numerous Russians' warmth and hospitality belied the other explanation, that totalitarianism had thoroughly dislodged Russians' abilities to form emotional connections. Understanding the specific historical configurations of power and disempowerment shaping workshop participants' responses offered an alternative means of explaining the Soviet and post-Soviet medicalization of reproduction. My analysis eventually focused on the disabling effects of provider deprofessionalization and patient disenfranchisement in a context where state discourses legitimated scientific authority over laypersons (an argument elaborated in Chapter 2). But the processes and outcomes of this project, including my simultaneous embrace of its values and discomfort with its methods of promoting them, seemed to exemplify the broader challenges of instrumentalizing feminist ideals in a global setting.[10] I have come to believe that feminist endeavors must incorporate both an expectation that "women's" interests can be marked by ruptures across time and space and a willingness to search for historically specific differences between our own experiences and those we hope to assist, before advising on change. Finally, feminist concerns to combat inequality and violence must deal honestly with the ethical dilemmas inherent in promoting change, both by listening to local voices and by reflexively addressing the potentials for coercion and abuse in our own deployment of power.

TWO

Stimulating Providers, Individualizing Labor

In WHO's Healthy Cities Project, and the projects affiliated with it, the promise of democratization for post-Soviet people involved first and foremost the creation of equity and empowerment for women, vis-à-vis health institutions and experts. I have argued that the agency's methods for promoting these valuable goals were inadequate for the task, for they neither incorporated local knowledge nor addressed the particular conditions shaping women's disempowerment in Russia. Nor did they consider how the legitimacy of notions of "democracy" and "equality" might be undermined when presented through a didactic, externally imposed training workshop. And still, though methodologically naive, WHO's concerns represented a position that has been all too rare in global and local efforts to engineer post-Soviet change. The agency's perspective that democracy should bring self-determination to the disenfranchised, should build equity rather than stratification, reflected the hopes of only a small minority of actors in the mid 1990s. For international lending agencies, local health care authorities, and many providers and patients themselves, improved health and well-being were to be pursued through privatizing strategies of accumulating wealth, despite the fact that—or even because—they would stratify Russian society.

Certain conceptual frames were persuasive to public health policymakers as they defined the problems of the Soviet health system and designed a path for reform. Highlighting an entirely distinct set of priorities than those advocated by WHO, Russian policymakers placed matters of financing at center stage while virtually excluding issues of community participation and democratization. The problems they identified and targeted for change drew on the neoliberal critique of the state that had become increasingly hegemonic in global policy circles and development institutions. Their goals were to decentralize and deregulate the Russian health care system, reorienting its financing and delivery methods on the basis of a market logic. Reformers favored the notion that health care should be a site of competition and consumption as a sharp contrast with the Soviet paradigm of social entitlements. They celebrated the improvements that would emerge when services were provided, priced, and appraised according to economic principles. Yet questions concerning the market's ability to serve collective social needs, and the state's obligation to monitor market practices in order to ensure fairness and effectiveness, were marginalized.

For observers and reformers committed to empowerment and equity in health care, a critical reading of the *Soviet* health care system is necessary that highlights both positive and constraining dimensions of the Soviet system that have otherwise received little attention in the dash toward markets, profits, and economic "rationalization." This is not, however, a proposal for a more "truly" socialist model of health care, a call for correcting "errors" in the Soviet version of a socialist welfare model and returning to a more "pure" form of socialist theory and practice. To dismantle the binary logic embedded in the Cold War imagination and move beyond a simplistic dichotomy between socialism as totalitarianism (or equality) and Western capitalism as freedom (or oppression) requires a radically new mode of inquiry (Gal and Kligman 2000a; Lampland 2002; Verdery 2002), one that Verdery has described as an analysis of the ways states of various kinds undertake "*practices of domination,* such as techniques of evangelizing, manipulations of time and space, modes of inscribing the . . . system on the bodies of its subjects" (Verdery 2002). The task is to ask how Soviet state power structured practices of domination in ways that were parallel to or distinct from techniques in Western contexts, while clarifying how the end of state socialism and introduction of market reforms has enabled new forms of domination to emerge.

As advocates writing in public health journals envisioned, market economics was to transform medical treatment into a consumer service, subject to the laws of supply and demand and the resulting "natural" processes of quality control that competition supposedly ensures. One of the most important effects of this new orientation was to occur in the moral quality of social relations. The introduction of market mechanisms in health care financing and delivery, reformers argued, would stimulate health workers and health care users to be more responsible, efficient, and ambitious in their goals. Individualized modes of change in the form of economic incentives aimed to motivate providers anew to continually improve their skills and the quality of care they offered. They would adopt an energetic, businesslike frame of mind and feel a sense of personal dignity. By extension, doctor-patient relations based on the profit motive would now exemplify consumer-producer interactions found in any other market sphere. This, it was thought, would increase providers' and consumers' responsibility and build trust between them. The promises of the market thus involved a new set of disciplinary mechanisms for individual persons, while setting the state free from most obligations of oversight, regulation, and intervention on behalf of citizens' interests. The unassailable logic of this argument in Russian policy circles was evident in the tactics of those critics who challenged market reforms and the withdrawal of government investments in health care. Generally, critics highlighted the importance of "fairness" by emphasizing the severe poverty of most Russians and their *inability* to pay for care: the virtue of a market logic per se for health care and the compromises it can create in patient care were barely discussed.

Rather than achieving the efficiency and rationality deemed absent in the Soviet model, the absence of strong regulatory procedures produced a bureaucratic paralysis when market reforms were introduced to St. Petersburg's health care system. With little oversight or surveillance, the St. Petersburg municipality, city insurance companies, and fund-holding intermediaries failed to ensure that the health care system had even the basic levels of funds and citizen protections.

MEDICINE, EMPOWERMENT, AND EQUITY: SOCIALIST IDEALS FOR HEALTH CARE REFORM

In the West, socialist theorists have outlined key principles essential for establishing empowerment and equity in health and medicine. Preventive and curative health care are part of a wider societal commitment to promoting the health of a population. Foremost in their approach is the equitable distribution of resources, including the basic material necessities for well-being: acceptable quality food, housing, education, and employment. Medicine is a component of this. In opposition to current trends in biomedicine that fragment the understanding of disease into single individuals, organs, or even genes, the emphasis in socialist medicine is to define ill health and disease in relation to political-economic inequalities, structural disparities, and insufficient resources. Thus, there is a critical recognition that public health indicators such as morbidity and mortality, life expectancy, and the prevalence of disease differ according to groups' socioeconomic resources and status in a given society. The recognition that ill health is a symptom of political-economic arrangements should lead the state and local communities to inquire why a particular disease or illness, disability or suffering, has befallen an individual or group; how social marginalization and inadequate access to resources caused or contributed to the illness, and how a rearrangement of structural resources may contribute to people's recovery and well-being.

Community participation in all aspects of health is also a necessary component of prevention, diagnosis, and treatment/recovery. Such participation extends from the level of organizing and mobilizing social groups for preventive care, to decision-making about treatment, including biomedical interventions. To make community participation feasible, individuals, neighborhoods, and communities must be organized into independent groups who can make demands on local and national governments, take responsibility for policy decisions about health-related matters, and undertake the work of implementing programs for their communities.

The priority placed on redistributing resources equitably and focusing on community participation has implications for the role of biomedical experts in the health process. Most notably, experts' authority to define and lead the policymaking process, as well as their monopoly over clinical decision-making, is diminished. Some socialist theorists, such as Vicente Navarro, have also advocated the deprofessionalization of medicine as a means of ending the class basis of relations between providers and patients. Moreover, socialist theorists hold cautious views on the use of technology in medicine: neither prioritized nor condemned, it is incorporated into a social model of care so that its value is consciously evaluated in terms of its ability to empower and increase individuals' well-being and control. This contrasts with mainstream biomedical practice, whose practitioners often prize technology in and of itself as symbolic of improved quality of care and subordinate patients' individual needs to it. Under socialist medicine, public health services would devote resources to improving prevention and primary care and ensuring access for rural and marginal populations, rather than developing urban-based high-tech specialized centers to treat disease. While the focus is on equity, socialist theorists strive to emphasize that tertiary care would not neglected in this model, either.[1]

The importance of the social and political-economic foundations of health was acknowledged by the World Health Organization in its 1978 Alma Ata Declaration. It was also a core principle of the Healthy Cities Project and informed the agency's calls for equity, as expressed in the slogan intended to drive public policies, "health for all." When St. Petersburg applied for membership in the Healthy Cities Project, it gave a commitment to the concepts of "health for all," a move that can only be seen as ironic in light of the fact that the city was—at the same time—engaged in the systematic dismantling of the comprehensive health care and welfare safety net created under the Soviet era.

SOVIET HEALTH CARE: A POLITICAL
INSTRUMENTALIZATION OF SOCIALIST IDEALS

In 1977 Vicente Navarro, a pioneering critic of medicine under capitalism, published an analysis of Soviet medicine and social security (Navarro 1977). Examining Soviet health care offered insights into why the existing model of socialism had failed to result in emancipatory outcomes for the masses, and many of his findings remain pertinent today. At the same time, Navarro's embrace of Marxist materialism prevented a similarly complex critique of the socialist ideal he proffered, and this model is unable to address certain dimensions of power and domination that emerged from the Soviet system's deprofessionalized structure of health care relations. In the analysis below, my description both draws on and amends Navarro's analysis to outline the modes of power and domination established by the Soviet health care system.

According to Navarro's socialist inquiry, the Soviet health care system was a hierarchically organized, bureaucratically administered, technology-based, and expert-centered curative model. The Bolsheviks established a universal free health care system characterized by a deprofessionalized cadre of medical workers, thus ending the class basis of health care and, supposedly, the exploitation of all workers entering the medical sphere. Yet Lenin's early visions that local committees comprising all interest groups (soviets) would gain the power to manage and administer welfare sectors, including health care, were quickly derailed. Membership in the Communist Party was the prerequisite for involvement in local soviets, so representatives of the health workers had a merely advisory role in the clinics and hospitals where they worked (Navarro 1977: 23–24). And following Lenin's death in 1924, instead of what is now called "community participation" Stalin instituted a rigid hierarchical model of top-down decision-making. The organizational structure and administration of Soviet health care services in place by 1936 modeled the bureaucratic hierarchicalization of all state sectors: supreme decision-making authority resided in the Ministry of Public Health, which reported to the Executive Committee of the Communist Party. Below the national ministry were ministries of health for each republic of the Soviet Union, and within republics, two administrative units were created (the *oblast'* and the *raion*) where local health departments managed the provision of health care. Chief administrators of all these levels were necessarily physicians, and their authority was rigidly graduated according to their place in the vertical hierarchy emanating from the Soviet Ministry of Public Health (Navarro 1977: 49). As a consequence of this structure, the lower levels of bureaucracy in the health care system were largely charged with the task of fulfilling orders from above, a situation that continued until the late 1980s.

The Party's centralized control and unwavering priority to industrialize the country resulted in a nationalized, bureaucratized health care system focused on increasing productivity. On-site medical and occupational health clinics known as the *"medsanchast'"* sector catered to state needs to ensure productivity through curative and preventive care. From the 1960s, these enterprise clinics conducted mass routine screening programs (Tulchinsky and Varavikova 1996), which were compulsory for all workers. Still, the structure of health care was highly divided and nucleated, separated according to the function and population group served, so that workers in high-productivity enterprises and Communist Party elites received distinct services from other groups.

This structure both resulted from and perpetuated the managerial character of medical care, in which the medical "expert" was the agent of action, and society, categorized and treated as "patients," was the passive object of expert care (Navarro 1977: 112). This emphasis on expertise and specialization (the Flexnerian model) was replicated within the health workers' labor force, with the hospital-based specialist granted more prestige than the generalist, and with all types of physicians enjoying higher social status and higher salaries than nurses and *feldshers*.[2] In maternity care, for example, midwives were restricted to auxiliary work, sewing tears and disposing of waste materials after the birth, but never conducting prenatal care or attending deliveries themselves. Among recipients of services, two categories of care existed: the general network (*obshchii set*) served the masses, whereas the restricted network (*zakritii set*) was provided for Party elites (Field 1957: 184–85). The vast majority of Soviet society used the general network of health care and may have had little knowledge that the other network even existed. Urban areas were substantially better funded than rural regions of the country (see also Ryan 1978).

Navarro cites three major developments in health and social services emerging from the state's prioritization of the more "productive" sectors of the labor force: (1) the development of separate and autonomous occupational health services administered by the management of industries rather than local soviets, intended to reduce workers' absenteeism; (2) the development of extensive child care centers to enable women's intensive participation in the work force;[3] and (3) the establishment of urban environmental health services to attack public health problems (Navarro 1977: 43).

State economic investments in health care—which was considered a "non-productive" sector relative to heavy industry and the military—further reflected these principles. Budget allocations to health care reached only about 3 percent of GDP (compared to 6.5–13 percent in Western countries); and a full 1 percent of this amount was devoted to the elite closed health care system (Barr and Field 1996: 308). Throughout the Soviet era, health care was funded through the residual principle, meaning that it was allocated "whatever was left over after other allocations had been made" (Field 1995: 1473–74; Sheiman 1995: 169). The average physician's salary was 10–15 percent lower than the average salary in the country, and remained the same regardless of the number of patients treated or the quality of care provided (Sheiman 1995: 170). This lower status in comparison with heavy industry entailed a leading cause of the feminization of the profession—70 percent of physicians in the Soviet Union were women (Navarro 1977: 79; Ryan 1978: 42–43; Schecter 1992a, b). The actual flows of funding were based on an extensive system, focusing on increasing the quantities of beds and numbers of physicians, rather than on intensive inputs for improved quality and equity. Hospitals were paid according to the number of beds filled, encouraging longer periods of hospitalization and extended expert control over patients.

In opposition to the egalitarian theories of socialist health care discussed above, which mandated comprehensive and equal levels of care across geographical areas, and despite the rhetoric of the Soviet regime, "it was Party policy that labor should be rewarded and taken care of in proportion to its productive input in the process of industrialization" (Navarro 1977: 46). Public health policies exploited the appearance of highly visible, accessible health care as a legitimating force for the state, while the actual quality of care for most of the population was poor and not equitable. Navarro critiques Soviet health care for failing to redefine medicine through socialist principles, citing the division of services into highly technical specialties, which both fragmented patient care and enabled an emphasis on experts' roles in defining and curing illness. He also raises the questionable critique that Soviet health care treated illness as a depoliticized, individualized concern (1977: 47–49). While the individual became a target of social control by some medical policies, such as the physical treatment of "deviant" sexual function (Kon 1995), in other cases (such as the aftermath of the Chernobyl explosion), the state created social categories of suffering and turned health care into a clearly politicized process (Petryna 2002).

DEMOCRATIZATION, DEPROFESSIONALIZATION, AND POWER IN THE SOVIET UNION AND RUSSIA

In contrast to the understanding of "democracy" as a matter of attitudes and behaviors advanced by WHO affiliates, Navarro's critique of the undemocratic character of the Soviet health care system provides a more comprehensive, structurally rooted vision of what a politicized, egalitarian social approach to health might entail. A cornerstone of his approach recognizes that the hierarchical, managerial, and technological structure of

Soviet health care stemmed from the centralization of power by the state and Party, to the exclusion of the masses of society.[4] Moreover, if lower-level Soviet bureaucrats had some degree of power, they were "ultimately subservient to the final and most powerful voice, the one of the top political structure" (Navarro 1977: 41). Critical of this structure and dedicated to the democratization and mass politicization of medicine, Navarro's study aims to advance a structural redistribution of power in society as a whole and within health care in particular.

Working from an ethnographic analysis of Soviet health care, however, I suggest that the concept of power informing Navarro's argument about deprofessionalization is constrained by its materialist vision. A key assumption in his study is that the deprofessionalization of medicine would result in a more equitable health care system—in other words, that eradicating the material form of inequality between providers and patients would effectively democratize health care and create equality in medicine. Yet the heightened focus on technology and expertise in Soviet medical education and public discourse, which Navarro discusses, constructed *symbolic* forms of inequality between health providers and patients based on the expert's possession of specialized knowledge. It is here that a reconsideration of the implications of deprofessionalization is necessary.

"Participation" for both health care users and workers was severely constrained during the Soviet era since policy decisions were made by the Ministry of Health in Moscow and fulfilled at the local levels by cadres whose authority was based on their membership in the Party. Ideologically, it was assumed that health care workers would have no interests separate from those of the Party; in practice, such an assumption neglected health workers' concerns and experiences, especially regarding their work conditions. With career advancement and access to policymaking linked to Party activism, doctors' "deprofessionalization" essentially meant disenfranchisement (Field 1991; Jones and Krause 1991; Krause 1991; Schecter 1992a, b). In contrast to the political-economic and social power enjoyed by organized professions in Western contexts (cf. Abbott 1988; Eckstein 1960; Freidson 1986 [1970], 1994), Soviet health care workers would more accurately be described as disenfranchised bureaucrats. In daily practice this social position meant that physicians were to defer to hospital administrators and public health authorities and had very narrow parameters for expressing professional autonomy.

Still, the regime's ideological emphasis on scientific expertise and technology led physicians to feel entitled to dominance and authority over laypersons. This contradictory approach to expertise—in which physicians were disenfranchised from political and economic power but constantly promoted as authorities with disciplinary power—resulted in a curious outcome. The clinic setting afforded physicians their sole arena for enacting professional authority (Field 1991). This was reflected in the terminology used—health care users were called "patients" [*bol'nye,* literally, "sick persons"] rather than users or consumers. Patients entering a clinic or hospital were to defer completely to expert authority.

Given this historical experience, it is questionable whether deprofessionalization by itself could have led to provider-patient "equality" outside of a locally accepted commitment to eliminating the symbolic authority associated with expert knowledge. Deprofessionalization combined with the emphatic, symbolic authority granted to expertise resulted in the systematic frustration of power and its expression in interpersonal interactions, not its erasure. Deprofessionalization strengthened physicians' commitment to medicalization, which essentially served as the primary means of realizing the power they were led to expect as medical specialists.

These paradoxical features of physicians' power were not readily visible to either Russians or outside observers. Seeking to promote "democratic" and egalitarian relations between Russian providers and patients in the early 1990s, WHO consultants assumed that Russian physicians' reluctance to accept their calls to increase women's autonomy reflected, in the words of one consultant, the tendency of "doctors everywhere" to "want to keep power for themselves." Unaware of the deprofessionalized structure of medicine and its constraints on physicians' "power," these consultants could not see that the hierarchical clinical interactions they witnessed might be the product of physicians' relative lack of power, the desperate weapons of those with a small bit of power turned against others with even less. Understanding this situation, we may argue that promoting "democracy" in health care would require restructuring the organization of the medical profession itself, to create the opportunities for physicians to pressure state policymakers and engage in dialogue with consumer groups— which themselves would need to be organized and empowered. Structurally based forms of political autonomy for health service users and providers—including physicians—could justifiably be seen as questions of "women's rights" and democracy in the post-Soviet era.

THE SOVIET ORGANIZATION OF MATERNAL HEALTH CARE

The resulting Soviet health system as experienced by ordinary citizens provided free primary care for all, based on residential areas; each neighborhood or area was a political unit called an *uchastok.* Within the *uchastok,* three independent branches of health care existed: general adult care, maternal and child care, and public health/environmental medicine.

There was no cooperative link between these three branches, which often provided their services in separate ambulatory polyclinics located within a given *uchastok*. These outpatient clinics provided referrals to the hospitals when inpatient care was deemed necessary; general hospitals, considered the secondary level of care, operated according to the district or *raion*, and served a larger proportion of the population than *uchastok* polyclinics. At the tertiary level of care were specialized hospitals devoted to specific illnesses such as TB, mental illness, and gynecological diseases. The notable implication of this fragmentation of services was the absence of continuity of care for patients. The responsibility for patients resided with the institution providing care, which switched with each episode of illness, or when outpatient treatment was converted to inpatient care and then back again.

Within the arena known as "maternal health," gynecological and obstetrical care were similarly divided into neighborhood outpatient clinics and maternity hospitals, and at the most specialized, tertiary level, gynecological hospitals. According to the chief doctor of one St. Petersburg maternity home, prior to 1988 maternity hospitals and women's consultation centers were structurally coordinated. Traces of this connection remained, as the first floors of several city maternity hospitals continued to house women's clinics that did not acquire their own freestanding buildings. However, the structural coordination was formally eliminated by the Public Health Committee in an effort to coordinate gynecological and pediatric care, a change that never fully materialized.[5] Since 1988, women in St. Petersburg attended one clinic for gynecological and prenatal care and gave birth in a maternity hospital staffed by completely different health care professionals. In the mid 1990s there were over forty women's clinics in St. Petersburg, located in every neighborhood. Women were eligible for free care at the clinic in the neighborhood of their official residence, but had to pay for services acquired at other clinics.[6] On the other hand, women were eligible for free childbirth services at any of the city's maternity hospitals. Women often entered the maternity hospital for the first time ever at the start of their labor, although many were admitted during the course of pregnancy for rest and observation. The lack of integration of pregnancy, birth, and general health care was criticized by virtually all maternal health professionals with whom I spoke; it exemplified the health care system's extreme focus on specialization, rather than on the health care needs of the community. It also reflected the narrow ways the Soviet state conceptualized women's health care, as merely the provision of abortions and management of pregnancy and childbirth.

The organization of care in maternity hospitals was further divided and nucleated, preventing any kind of continuous relationship with a single caregiver or group of caregivers even within the birth experience.

Providers were assigned to one of three wards of the hospital—the gyneco-logical/prenatal ward, the labor and delivery ward, or the postnatal ward. Physicians were thus responsible solely for the limited segment of care they gave, and any one patient would likely be under the care of at least three different physicians who were structurally separate from each other. Importantly, however, physicians on the prenatal and postnatal wards worked shifts in the labor and delivery wards about six times a month to maintain their skills for birth.

In addition to physicians' political and economical disenfranchisement and low pay, the fractured structure of patient care directly impeded physicians' ability to experience themselves as fully authoritative, responsible professionals. Doctors I worked with called the division of maternity care into distinct prenatal, postnatal, and delivery rooms, in which patients were shuffled through the hospital with a maximum degree of discontinuous, fragmented care, a guarantee of "collective irresponsibility" [*kollektivnaia bezotvetstvennost'*].

FROM DEPROFESSIONALIZATION TO PRIVATIZATION: A GLOBAL REFORM AGENDA FOR HEALTH

The types of "problems" I have highlighted thus far—citizens' lack of voice in either their health care or their professional lives, the disempowerment created by a bureaucratized, top-down decision-making system, and the lack of equality, were not the problems identified as most pressing to elites who would direct Russia's post-Soviet health reforms. In the immediate aftermath of the collapse of the Soviet Union, the International Monetary Fund, the World Bank, and USAID, along with bilateral development agencies in Western Europe, promoted a neoliberal program of "shock therapy" and structural adjustment to transform Russia's command economy based on centralized planning into a liberal, deregulated economy based on the laws of the market. Privatization, liberalization, and deregulation were the three components of this policy highlighted by enthusiastic reformers in these institutions and within Russia itself. They sought to replace centralized price controls with market mechanisms so that the production and distribution of consumer products would occur through the laws of supply and demand. Privatization would offer producers incentives to work efficiently in sync with market signals, meeting consumer needs. Another central component of the privatization process involved dismantling the comprehensive Soviet system of social guarantees, from employment and housing to health care and education. By withdrawing state subsidies and drastically reducing public spending, economists aimed to bring inflation under control and stimulate a complacent Russian labor force to work harder (Field, Kotz, and Bukhman 2000: 164).

Analyses of the effects of these reforms are inherently political. The World Bank's analysis, "Transition-The First Ten Years: Analysis and Lessons for Eastern Europe and the Former Soviet Union" (2002) acknowledges that economic liberalization has had negative effects on social safety nets. Yet its focus remains firmly rooted in the need for "discipline and encouragement" (2002: 81), by which is meant reducing state expenditures and targeting assistance only to the most needy sectors of society. The 149-page booklet has a sole 7-page chapter detailing social welfare issues; in that space it attempts to address reforms of the region's pension systems, cash assistance benefits, education, and health care—the latter of which is briskly covered in less than one page. A key piece of advice given for improving educational and health care services is for governments to transfer resources from personnel to infrastructures and materials; apparently, providing teachers and health care providers with a basic living wage does not constitute what the World Bank considers addressing "the most vulnerable, such as those affected by the increase in utility prices and by the labor shedding resulting from hard budget constraints on enterprises" (2002: 81). The International Monetary Fund has been even less concerned with social welfare; its measurements of reform "progress" are limited to the level of privatization and GNP, while ignoring levels of poverty, equity in income distribution, and the contribution of "growth" to the standard of living of the poor (Krueger 2002). In this logic, the 1998 decision to devalue the ruble, which resulted in the losses of savings for millions of Russians, is simply lauded as a sign of Russian authorities' "virtue," "long-standing courage and persistence," despite "painful" periods (Krueger 2002: 1). The roles of government officials in disenfranchising the vast majority of Russian people, by usurping public resources themselves and allowing their accumulation by a small number of oligarchies, remains conveniently ignored (Cohen 2001; Field, Kotz, and Bukhman 2000: 166).[7]

Also missing from these reports is that the vast majority of Russians have experienced market-based reforms as profound economic dislocation, vulnerability, and insecurity. In the first stages of privatization and the lifting of price controls, factories closed down or stopped paying wages, while prices for basic necessities soared. Employees who retained their jobs in state bureaucratic sectors found that the wages they received would now barely cover the costs of a modest food budget. Subsidies for housing and transportation were being substantially reduced, and previously free services such as health care and education now required payments. By 1995 the value of the average real wage was only 51 percent of its 1991 value, while the real value of the minimum monthly pension had fallen to a mere 40 percent of its 1991 value (Field, Kotz, Bukhman 2000: 165). Moreover, the quality of public services decreased substantially. There was no funding for infrastructural repairs, and basic necessities such as textbooks in schools and sheets in hospitals had to be subsidized by citizens. Scholarly analyses that acknowledge these effects offer alternative views of structural adjustment:

> Price liberalization produced rapid inflation, rather than an efficient re-allocation of production. The cuts in state spending and the rigorously tight monetary policy contributed to the severe depression and denied needed funds to Russian enterprises seeking to modernize. Hasty privatization turned state enterprises over to influential insiders but produced no improvement in business performance. Demolishing the social safety net left individuals bereft of any security, and the expected "work incentives" were irrelevant, given the absence of employment opportunities in the collapsing economy. (Field, Kotz, and Bukhman 2000: 166)

While a small segment of the population has benefited tremendously from privatization, the effects of neoliberal reforms have been devastating to the vast majority of ordinary Russians. Overlapping directly with the implementation of structural adjustment policies beginning in 1992 were drastic rises in mortality from alcoholism, cardiovascular disease, violence, and trauma—all linked to prolonged and severe stress. And while Western apologists for structural adjustment policies explain rising mortality through such victim-blaming arguments as the Russian penchant for vodka (Eberstadt 1999), it is rather obvious that the massive social dislocation and economic deprivation created by shock therapy have contributed to Russia's serious health crisis. The celebratory discourses of the IMF and minimal attention paid to poverty by the World Bank suggest that Western agendas for privatization have been systematically divorced from concern with the "*concrete human costs*—the acute physical and psychological suffering and the catastrophic regression in public health" that these policies have engendered (Field, Kotz, and Bukhman 2000: 172).

NEOLIBERAL REFORMS IN RUSSIAN HEALTH CARE

Between 1993 and 1994, the same period that WHO was actively encouraging the St. Petersburg Public Health Committee to commit itself to the principles of equity and social well-being as a "healthy city," health planners throughout Russia were deeply involved in a very different kind of reform agenda. Following the advice of the World Bank and proponents of neoliberal health care systems, they undertook fundamental transformations in the centrally planned, universal, free health care system. The key goal was to shift the funding of health care from the government budget to an insurance-based system, which would involve deregulation and the introduction of market mechanisms to promote "cost-effectiveness." The creation of an insurance mechanism as a means of increasing funding had been pursued since 1988, before the demise of the Soviet system. Yet it gained extensive momentum in the early 1990s, and legislation for a universal obligatory medical insurance system was finalized in 1993. It decentralized policymaking by delegating authority to regional administrations, charging them with developing their own insurance-based mechanism. Commenting on the consequences of this decentralization, Judyth Twigg observed that by the late 1990s, there were eighty-nine different health care systems in the eighty-nine regions of the Russian Federation (2000: 48).

The goals of the insurance system were to provide additional sources of revenue outside the government budget and to introduce market-based efficiency, competition, and provider-incentives to stimulate work (Twigg 2000: 44). Ideally, an insurance system was also intended to promote competition, as providers of services (hospitals and clinics) competed with each other for contracts with insurance companies, and as insurance companies competed among themselves. Additional reforms were to include a shift in emphasis away from expensive hospital care to primary care and outpatient care as cost-saving measures. Funds for this system were to flow from a 3.6 percent payroll tax exacted from all employers and a governmental contribution on behalf of the nonworking population. By levying a tax specifically for health care, the state sought to increase funds and ensure that certain resources would be earmarked only for medical and preventive services; yet practical actions taken by local administrations in the first decade of reforms demonstrate that the primary goal has been to withdraw the state from involvement in health care, to exempt it from the responsibility of ensuring that all members of the population have access to health care. The details of these reforms and specific experimentation processes in different regions have been analyzed in numerous studies (Curtis, Petukhova, and Taket 1995; Shchepin 2000; Sheiman 1995; Twigg 2000, 2002). My goal below is to examine the ideological concepts and debates that shaped the reform context and prioritized individual and interpersonal change and the delegitimation of equity, rather than a collective responsibility for the health and well-being of all citizens.

Throughout the 1990s, Russian scholarly journals of public health became a public arena for policymakers and researchers to trumpet the benefits of nongovernmental, commercial enterprises in health care. Almost without ever questioning the suitability of market mechanisms for improving health outcomes, the problems identified with the Soviet health-care system—inertia, rigidity, a top-down planning process, lack of financing, no "stimulus" for work, a lack of trust between patients and providers, the lack of responsibility by providers—were portrayed as readily solved by the panacea of market economics (Golukhov, Shilenko, and Shilenko 1996: 25; Ovcharov and Shchepin 1996: 26; Togunov 1999). Competition between institutions and economic stimuli for increasing providers' productivity were assumed to lead automatically to improvements in quality of care. Quite often, the market was hailed with unbridled enthusiasm as the necessary and sufficient solution.

Organizing the provision of health care on the basis of a market logic involved fundamental reconceptualizations of the participants in the health care sphere, their roles and interactions. Provider-patient relations were now to be understood as analogous to those of producers and consumers in all other areas of market exchange; providers would act as producers [*proizvoditeli*] of market services [*meditsinskikh uslug*], and patients were to be understood as consumers [*potrebiteli uslug*], not patients [*bol'nye*] (Togunov 1999: 1). As in all other areas of consumer activity, consumer demand was to be the driving force of health care provision, with services subject to the flexible pricing mechanism associated with supply and demand (Golukhov, Shilenko, and Shilenko 1996: 28; Grigor'ev 1995: 49). In this context, reformers assumed that the possibility of economic compensation would motivate producers of health care services to constantly improve the quality of the product they offer. They would become "interested" in an economic sense in their work and seek to raise their qualification level, increase the volume of their productivity, and assume greater responsibility for their work (Kudrin and Leizerman 2002: 18; Ovcharov and Shchepin 1996: 25–26). Key to the market's perceived promise for catalyzing needed changes was the transformation it was expected to create in individual personalities and behaviors of health care workers:

> The market opens up the same conditions and opportunities for everyone everywhere. Under such conditions, one feels more qualified, energetic, you consider yourself a talented specialist. The market is profitable to those who want and are able to work and live well. It is a true sign of civilization—not only the level of material civilization, but also the person's cast of mind—business-like, energetic, and able to predict the future. (Grigor'ev 1995: 49)

In language hauntingly reminiscent of early Soviet discourses on creating a "New Soviet Man," reformers argued that "fulfilling the demand for quality and effective medicine is not only a matter of structural and organizational transformations. The first and most difficult task involves forming the personality of the 'new' worker." This ambitious and capable personality would be focused on the clear-cut, precise goals of enhancing productivity and ensuring "the rational use of production resources," would be founded on "self-discipline, responsibility for one's work, a feeling of personal dignity, and aspirations for professional perfection" (Kudrin and Leizerman 2001: 18). Some persons, it was claimed, were fortunate to already have this personality type, and their achievements were being rightfully earned: "Success comes to those who orient themselves first, objectively evaluate the situation, make the right decisions, and take actions" (Grigor'ev 1995: 49). Others, however, would need to be taught, or, in the view of one article, properly "managed." This argument construed the problems in health care provision as issues of management and interpersonal relations. Stimulating workers' productivity through economic incentives and appropriate social management techniques would work to transform health care workers' personalities, behaviors, and interpersonal relations:

> The search for a stimulus for work is especially relevant today, and a mechanism for work motivation is needed, founded on a strict correspondence between salary and the worker's investment in his work. We must build a social, motivational orientation to management. However, it is currently extremely difficult to establish positive changes, since the systematic crisis Russian society is experiencing has, at its base, a crisis of management, which, already long ago, turned into *a crisis of human relations [krizis upravleniia, kotoryi uzhe davno prevratilsia v krizis chelovecheskikh otnoshenii]*." (Kudrin and Leizerman 2001: 19; italics added)

The crisis, in these authors' view, was the "deeply deformed" [*gluboko porazhennoi*] relations of production. To ensure that an effective social management could be undertaken by administrators, government must "stay out" of the process. Market incentives alone, it was thought, will enable pioneering physicians to improve health care:

> Clearly, a condition for the success of such reforms is the withdrawal of government from primary care [*razgosudarstvlenie*]. . . . An independent primary care doctor [integrated in the public health system] for whom specific economic stimuli have been developed, is the most important, dynamic link of the reforms, able to radically raise the quality of medical assistance. (Zel'kovich 1996: 38)

Similarly, the introduction of users' fees was promoted as leading patients to become more responsible for their health (Lindenbraten and Gololobova 2002: 23). Yet there was little interest in cultivating a sense of "responsibility" among the population that involved establishing and actively promoting patients' rights, authority, and participation in clinical decisions. While the concept of patients' rights has gained some credibility in legislative circles, its perceived importance has not been sufficient enough to persuade policymakers to establish limits and controls on the market, or even to establish a mechanism for protecting citizens' rights. It was only in July 1998—five years after the legislation approving an insurance-based financing system went into effect—that the Russian Ministry of Health, the federal Compulsory Medical Insurance Fund, and the State Standardizing Agency, Gosstandart, developed an official standardization system for health services. Still, as late as 2000, one observer of patients' rights acknowledged, "No action has been adopted at the Federal level which outlines the legal bases for a system of various bodies and establishments to carry out [the] protection of the lawful interests of the citizens" regarding the provision of medical care that is appropriate in volume and quality (Tsyboulsky 2001: 261). The general assumption among public health experts was that provider authority needed to be strengthened, not reduced (Perepletchikov 1994)—and this view had worked its way into earlier drafts of patients' rights legislation since the mid 1980s (Tsyboulsky 2001: 261). Some authors even advocated direct payment for services as a means of helping reestablish the doctor's authority (Ovcharov and Shechepin 1996: 26).

The idea of privatizing *all* health care was not supported; even the most avid proponents of neoliberal reforms recognized the need to maintain a government system of universal health care that would serve the most impoverished residents (Golukhov, Shilenko, and Shilenko 1996: 26; Ovcharov and Shechepin 1996; Pogorelov and Chudinova 1996: 42; Pokrovskii, Shchepin, Ovcharov, and Nechaev 1995: 5). This fact alone suggests an implicit recognition of the market's limited abilities to serve the public good. Yet innovation, creativity, and development were seen as the sole property of the market. A stratified system of services offering different levels of quality was the implicit and sometimes explicit principle of reform; in other words, the reorganization of health care services on the basis of *inequity* became seen as a necessary and moral development. Experts claimed that those consumers willing and able to pay have the right to the availability of superior quality services:

> The creation and development of a non-governmental sector of paid medical services . . . is objectively necessary because of the deep differentiation of consumer demand of different groups and strata of the population and the poor effectiveness of the existing governmental structure of service. . . . Global experience shows that high income groups of citizens prefer medical services in the non-governmental sector for being more qualified, offering a higher level of service, and the right to choose the doctor and medical institutions. (Golukhov, Shilenko, and Shilenko 1996: 25–26)

The key concept here is that of "consumer demand"—those persons able and willing to pay have been transformed from patients into consumers, buyers who demand high quality, nongovernmental services. Implicitly, this excerpt suggests that the health care interests of nonconsumer citizens are of little importance. Fulfilling consumer demand was the name of the game. Even critics of fee-for-service and private medicine objected not to the market principle per se, but to the practical inability of the majority of persons to pay for care. Their articles tended to be written as reminders not to neglect the poor masses, without suggesting that economic incentives in and of themselves could have negative effects on health outcomes. Such arguments for "fairness" and equity were in the minority, and generally served to alert readers to the devastation being wrought by ignoring the needs of the masses of people. One article, for example, highlighted how "stratification can reach catastrophic proportions inasmuch as economic programs and actual measures are oriented to the rich and not to the general masses of the population" (Pogorelov and Chudinova 1996: 42). Another cited statistics comparing the substantially lower levels of government expenditures for public health in Russia (2.2 percent of GDP, with that in Germany (8.2 percent,) the U.S. (13 percent), and Great Britain (5.9 percent), and highlighted the fact that state funding of health care in Russia declined by 33 percent between 1991 and 1998. "In this way, the population of Russia has had to compensate for the reduction in government funding of public health at their own expense with their own resources" (Maksimova and Gaenko 2001: 10). Still, even when critiquing the state's neglect and hypocrisy vis-à-vis the majority of citizens, these authors did not launch a frontal attack on market ideology or propose concrete policy alternatives. They tended to insist that governments facilitate people's "adaptation to the new economic conditions" (Pogorelov and Chudinova 1996: 41), and accepted the notion that "individual responsibility" for one's health needed to be cultivated. One article tacitly acknowledged this while encouraging the government to make such steps possible: "The average salary at present does not enable a typical Russian family to stop relying on free services and government entitlements in such important spheres as housing, education, medicine, vacation, and to accept full financial responsibility" for their lives (1996: 42).

For proponents of the market logic, however, arguments for "fairness" as equity were unconvincing; some authors went as far as to assert that a utilitarian logic based on economic returns represented the new, necessary moral basis of service provision:

Arguments against the development of the non-governmental sector of public health based on "fairness" in the provision of citizens' medical care, or arguments that the notion of economic order is inappropriate when speaking of health as a higher good do not consider a series of important issues. First of all, the potential for health is a substantial part of national wealth and must be examined as an economic category. Resources for its protection, support, and renewal are limited. The use of resources must provide for the protection of the population's health in light of economic return [*s uchetom ekonomicheskoi otdachi*]. (Golukhov, Shilenko, and Shilenko 1996: 25–26)

In a logic that ironically reproduced the Soviet privileging of industrially productive sectors of the population, market reformers viewed economically successful members of society as deserving of resources, while portraying others as a drain on the nation's vitality. This vision found its way into some Russian research on health care reform, too. An inquiry into which social groups were paying for health care and how much they were paying concluded that "the working population pays more than most impoverished groups" (Lindenbraten and Gololobova 2002: 23), as if to suggest that the poorest members of society were not forced to pay significant amounts of money for care. Yet the study compared amounts only in absolute terms, without considering the amounts that various payments represented in proportion to people's incomes. Nor did it inquire whether the lack of payment might indicate that these groups lacked services altogether or accessed only a substandard quality of care.

The likelihood that providers might withhold treatment or engage in unnecessary medical interventions to earn additional income was rarely acknowledged in these debates, and even when the possibility of such practices was mentioned, no precise policy measures were proposed to protect patients. The phrasing of one article that did comment on this issue is telling:

> The specific character of the doctor-patient relationship involves the potential for creating superfluous demand; there is also a possibility for doctors to make covert, corporate deals with pharmaceutical companies. It is widely known, for example, that over-diagnosis and over-treatment was widespread among American surgeons in the 1970s and '80s. Such practices led to a significant rise in profits for private clinics as a result of higher prices for services without appropriate therapeutic effect. Corporate unification can restrain price competition on the pharmaceutical market and impede raising the quality of medical services for citizens. (Golukhov, Shilenko, and Shilenko 1996: 27)

This acknowledgment that an economic basis for clinical decisions can lead to abuses by providers—one of the few references to such problems in the Russian public health literature from the mid 1990s—is notably vague and dismissive, as if the cases of overtreatment largely occurred in another time and place and no longer posed serious threats. The article did not proceed to discuss modes of regulation or control to ensure that the quality of patient treatment would not be compromised by economic incentives; indeed, it changed the topic altogether to discuss the need for strengthening physician authority.

Swept away by an almost blind enthusiasm for the need to make profitability the driving motivation of health care workers, policymakers defined a major problem with the Soviet system to be the fact that workers had no incentives to improve their performance. Because doctors earned the same amount of money regardless of the quality and volume of their work, they claimed that the system had built-in disincentives for health providers to do anything more than the absolute minimum, to improve their skills, or to feel committed to their profession. Constructing human motivation through a model of *Homo economicus,* they argued that economic incentives, virtually by themselves, would provide the answer to substandard health care. Payments would directly (mechanistically) motivate physicians to raise their qualifications, increase their effectiveness, and lead workers to become "interested" in the outcomes of their performance. Of course, this assumption reduced the complex motivations and interests driving physicians to a single concern with monetary compensation. Like the justifications for neoliberal health care reforms documented throughout much of Europe, this approach failed to recognize the myriad kinds of "interests" and "stimuli" health professionals hold, such as "a sense of duty, pride in one's work, compassion, a desire to be useful or make a difference, a desire to be current versus becoming a has-been, a desire to be liked or respected or in demand or a sense of affiliation" (Light 1995: 152).

Such arguments placed enormous faith in the ability of an unregulated market to solve human problems, while viewing governments as merely hopeless sites for poor productivity and inefficiency (Light 1995: 152). Thus, a key term in this literature was *razgosudarstvlenie,* the withdrawal of government or the disinvestment of government. Advocates for market-based reforms ignored the fact that tying clinical decisions to physicians' remuneration may both conflict with patients' health needs and undermine alternative motivations for practicing medicine. If health care workers' personalities had been dulled by the systemic lack of "stimuli," then introduction of an economic logic to their work was expected to make them more responsible, effective, and active. Key to this transformation was competition, portrayed as an almost magical property of market systems that made actors "dynamic" and stimulated them to strive, aspire, and succeed—it was assumed—to improve patients' health.

This magical market property of competition was discussed as if existing outside larger economic and social frameworks. Authors failed to recognize that when faced with competition, providers may find alternative responses that do not require them to become more productive or efficient. They may search for easier or more profitable solutions to deal with the presence of competitors. They may specialize to create a market niche, innovate to create new demands, expand diagnosis and treatment to increase revenues, or refuse to treat costly or burdensome patients (Light 1995: 146). While not all of these developments would necessarily lead to harmful outcomes for patients, neither do they automatically lead to cost-effective care or the protection of patients' interests. Studies of public health in the U.S. and Western Europe have found that for competition to function effectively (in other words, to improve quality of care and lower costs), several important preconditions must be in place. There must be a well-informed consumer base, transparency regarding the supply, and an effective regulatory system to ensure that incentives do not compromise care and lead to abuse. In health care, what consumers buy are interventions, and additional medical interventions may not be necessary or beneficial for patients' health. Competition without regulation, transparency, and an informed consumer base creates the conditions for exploitation and compromises in patient care. Indeed, in contexts where the importance of health as a social good has been recognized, government control has not disappeared; it has been transformed. Instead of offering direct inputs in care provision, states often take on a supervisory role, ensuring close oversight of the market. "The greater the level of market-style incentives that the country's policymakers introduce, and the more decentralized management the health system has, then the greater the regulatory role of the State if the citizenry is to receive a consistent, universally accessible standard of care" (Saltman 2002: 1681). It is not surprising, therefore, that achieving high-quality care in a market system does not occur automatically if the state merely recedes from activity. Achieving improved quality through market mechanisms requires extensive public resources (Saltman 2002: 1681–82).

Yet advocates of a market logic for health services in Russia offered little specific discussion of how to assess quality and effectiveness of care. It is not clear how the establishment of economic incentives would lead to better health outcomes in cases where physicians had an incentive to provide cheaper or more profitable care, rather than good quality care, which may involve fewer technological interventions or medicines, for example. Still, Russian critics of market-based services have been unable either to critique theories and practices of privatization or to offer precise ways of ensuring that an orientation toward profit-making in health care delivery and financing would not have negative effects on either the poor or the wealthy.[8]

ST. PETERSBURG'S HEALTH CARE REFORMS: DEREGULATE, DIVEST, DECEIVE

St. Petersburg city authorities made no overt decision to eliminate universal free health care. The establishment of the health insurance system was intended to improve the quality of care while ensuring increased revenues and more efficient use of resources. All official residents of St. Petersburg were covered by compulsory medical insurance (Curtis 1997: 673). In practice, however, the additional funding for health care intended in insurance-based plans did not materialize. As in experiments throughout Russia, neither employers nor local governments fulfilled their financial obligations to the insurance funds, with governments in particular paying less than their obligatory share (Twigg 2000: 46). In St. Petersburg, insurance systems were organized as territorial medical organizations (TMOs) responsible for a specific region of the city's population, and served as fund-holders for these payroll taxes and government funds (Curtis 1997; Sheiman 1995; Zel'kovich 1996). Yet much of the money that did arrive in the TMOs got "stuck" there, and did not effectively get to the clinics as intended (Zel'kovich 1996: 38). In 1997, the health insurance funds in all of Russia collected only 37.5 percent of the total needed to finance the "free health care" officially established under the compulsory medical insurance program (Twigg 2000: 47). As a result, health care institutions were chronically and severely underfunded and had insufficient medications, irregular access to hot water, and no resources for structural repairs. Moreover, competition between insurance companies or providers was hardly established. Patients were still assigned to clinics based on their place of residence (leaving them no choice in their primary health care providers). Nor did insurance companies compete with each other as purchasers of health care from hospitals and polyclinics, for they divided up the city's providers among themselves, effectively eliminating competition (Curtis et al. 1997: 679; Twigg 2000: 50). Moreover, the incentive system supposed to encourage cost effectiveness was structured at the level of the clinic, not individual physicians. To deal with the lack of resources, physicians increasingly had to ask patients to bring needed medications and even bed sheets. For the vast majority of health care workers, salaries remained barely above the minimum standard of living. In 1998 health care financing from both government and employer expenditures declined by 18 percent from the levels in 1997 (Twigg 2000: 60), and following the economic crash in August, the Russian government proposed revising the list of covered services as well as reducing the payroll tax from 3.6 to 3.4 percent (Twigg 2000: 53, 61). Confronting this problem, both the IMF (Dmitriev et al. 2000) and World Bank (1996: 36) advocated rewriting the listed of covered services under the compulsory medical insurance to fit the actual available budget—in other words, to eliminate promises and expectations of a universal system of health care.

The guiding principles shaping the reform policies of the St. Petersburg Public Health Committee involved a commitment not to equity and social justice, but to the development of markets and an economic logic for health care provision. This ideological position was expressed in several areas of policy. The committee emphasized the need for patients to contribute financially to the costs of health care. Asserting plans to ensure that 8–10 percent of the total volume of medical services would be paid for through out-of-pocket users' fees, the Public Health Committee justified this change as promoting the moral responsibility of citizens: "This principle is widespread throughout the entire civilized world: the patient's responsibility for taking care of his/her own health significantly increases when some medical services are paid completely or partially, by the patient himself" (Public Health Committee 1994: 8).

The move to reduce hospitalization rates and lengths of stay was driven by the high cost of tertiary-level care, not a commitment to promote patients' autonomy or a focus on prevention. As in contexts throughout Europe (Light 1995, 2000), it was accompanied by the deregulation of health care quality, which led to reductions in both equity and access to health care by the poor. For example, to reduce hospitalization rates, the city municipality introduced financial incentives for outpatient treatment and penalties for providers who failed to act "cost-effectively." This required a set of standards and evaluative criteria for assessing "effective treatment."[8] Creating such criteria proved a difficult task, and in St. Petersburg as throughout Russia, the process was beset by the pervasive danger that economic incentives would compromise patients' interests. Although recognizing that conflicts of interest could arise, the St. Petersburg Public Health Committee was reluctant to establish regulatory measures on providers and insurance companies. The committee's 1994 official statement of its health care reform agenda alluded to the need to guard against allowing economic interests to diminish the provision of quality treatment, asserting that criteria for quality of care should be based on medical standards alone, not "medical-economic standards" (1994: 20). The text went on to discuss how monitoring health care institutions' treatment decisions was to be the work of expert commissions based in insurance companies, highly qualified medical specialists whose salaries were not to depend on their decisions. And yet, the same text nonetheless suggests that economic criteria would indeed be made central to health care decision-making. The insurance company's expert commissions were to establish a protocol that included assessments of the necessity of diagnostic and treatment services *from the point of view of expenditures.* "In sum, the work of the expert is to create numerical scores and findings regarding the responsibility of medical institutions. We are talking, of course, about economic responsibility" (1994: 21). No mention of patients' interests followed.

St. Petersburg health care experts in the mid 1990s felt that these reforms had led to a situation in which "norms for provision levels were being eroded and . . . the new system had no effective mechanism to ensure that provision across the region would be kept above minimum acceptable levels" (Curtis et al. 1997: 682). While insurance companies were working to establish guidelines and criteria for quality and "cost-effective" care, there was no clear-cut system for monitoring the insurance companies and defending patients' rights. In one study of health care reforms throughout the Russian Federation, St. Petersburg outpatient clinics were cited as having impeded appropriate hospital admissions due to the system of economic incentives (Sheiman 1995: 178). Health providers in St. Petersburg were taken into account only as economic agents who mechanistically react to economic motivations; their social and political roles were virtually ignored. Health care users were also excluded as agents —let alone decision-makers—in health care policy: they were transformed into consumers with demands to be fulfilled for profit. They had no choice in primary care provider, nor did they have input into which insurance agency purchased their health care (Curtis et al. 1997: 673). (Fortunately, they did have a choice of maternity hospital, though not prenatal care clinic.) At the center of reforms were insurance companies and the TMO fund-holders, for they were considered to have the "economic motivation to choose the most efficient units" (Sheiman 1995: 178–79).

In a statement describing the main goals for developing government regulation in public health for the decade of 2000–2010, an author's collective led by Academician Shchepin of the Russian Academy of Medical Sciences acknowledged that the government had failed to articulate a clearly defined policy for ensuring citizens' access to high-quality medical care during the rapid privatization process. Extensive structural unevenness in quality and availability of care, and the rise of a shadow market in public health, were the results. They advocated that the accessibility of medical services needed to be placed at the ideological and organizational core of government policies, and should include a systematized approach to the provision of free medical care and a clear delineation of services where user fees should be established. In particular, they suggested that all citizens should be guaranteed an equal and equally accessible level of primary medical care, while the availability of specialized, high-quality care should be rationed by type of disease and population group. The provision of free medical care, they claimed, must be insured particularly for rural populations, women and children, the elderly, and the disabled (Shchepin 2000: 7). Unfortunately, by the time this statement was issued, the level and quality of free health care in Russia had declined dramatically; it was widely assumed that fee-for-service care was the only way to ensure basic supplies and decent treatment.

In ideological terms, the state represented its encouragement of users' fees not primarily as its own withdrawal from service provision but as a moral process of stimulating health care workers to become motivated and productive and encouraging citizens to take "individual responsibility" for their health. Both of these goals relied on a logic of individualizing and privatizing forms of change in explicit contrast to visions of collective responsibility and participation. Reformers never considered the government's responsibilities to facilitate people's active, informed participation in their own health care and professionals' rights to organize for workplace interests. To do so would require broader understanding of human motivations and greater investments in economic, legal, and social kinds of reform than necessary when analyzing the problem through the narrow logic of neoliberal economics alone. It would require structuring transparency in institutions' quality, outcomes, and pricing, promoting the actual realization of patients' rights as a cultural value and systemic requirement, and making transparent grievance procedures accessible for all. Instead of undertaking any of these innovations, the state failed to fulfill even its own diminished obligation to contribute fully on behalf of the nonemployed sectors, allowing the already poor conditions of free health care to become further aggravated. Physicians and laypersons alike considered policymakers incorrigibly remiss in their obligations to provide an acceptable level of health care. Some were outraged at "the bureaucrats" who "do nothing for women's health," while others' anger expressed itself through a resigned cynicism about the state's ineptitude and indifference toward common people.

THREE

Individualizing Disciplines of Sex Education

As we have seen, projects to cure the pathologies of Russian women's health ranged widely, depending on who diagnosed the disease. WHO consultants highlighted institutions' disregard for women's autonomy, rights, and choice in childbirth. They encouraged providers to accept new values and behaviors that enacted "democratic" principles in the clinic. Global and local policy reformers emphasized the absence of economic stimuli for health workers, which they believed discouraged providers from ensuring quality treatment. Their projects introduced a model of consumer relations in health care to reward economic "rationality" and stimulate competitiveness. In the process, they too hoped to modify workers' clinical behaviors and reshape their personalities.

In contrast with these experts, clinic doctors defined the most glaring arenas of crisis to be women's poor health, ignorance, and apathy toward their condition. In interviews, they emphasized widespread complications during pregnancy, frequent birth traumas in newborns, an abortion rate that was double the birth rate, and explosive rates of sexually transmitted infection.[1] Doctors felt that working in reproductive health entailed stemming the tides of catastrophe, with ever-waning resources. An oft-cited proverb—"drowning victims must pull themselves out with their own hands"—captured the sense of abandonment providers felt at the state's failures to preserve social welfare. Yet when asked to explain the causes of these problems, providers tended to focus on women themselves. They acknowledged that poverty aggravates illness; they recognized, for example, that high food costs and low salaries can result in poor nutrition and anemia. But their critiques targeted young people's social and moral deficits. Providers repeatedly cited the population's "low level of culture" [*kul'turnost'*] and an underdeveloped sense of individual character [*lichnost'*] as causes of poor health. In this way, they shared the tendency of policymakers to target the self for moral transformations.

The pursuit of moral personhood shaped health education work in St. Petersburg's clinics in the mid 1990s. As an example of efforts to heal Russian society physically, socially, and spiritually, it struck me as curious that these projects largely disregarded the historical and political-economic factors that contributed to Russians' poor sexual and reproductive health. In 1990s Chile, by contrast, health promoters working with poor, disadvantaged, and vulnerable sectors emphasized the economic and social dimensions of the health risks people faced. In this way, their tactics critically opposed government-sponsored campaigns that defined "personal responsibility" as the main strategy for ensuring health, and they empowered residents to make demands on the state (Paley 2001). In Russia, too, I saw political-economic causes of ill health that seemed important to discuss in educational frameworks. The widespread use of abortion was a prime example. A practice rooted in the early decades of the Soviet era, it reflected historical constraints of Soviet pro-natalism and state production priorities, rather than the simple "choice" of Russian women seeking to control their fertility. The Soviet public health system institutionalized abortion as the most accessible means of fertility control.[2] Provided by (mostly women) physicians who earned meager salaries, abortions were more convenient for the state than researching, developing, or importing contraceptives (Popov 1992). Official ideology opposed abortion and continually exhorted women to increase childbearing. Clearly, abortion use was not simply a matter of individual, rational (or irrational, "uncultured") choices, but reflected a structured outcome of a specific political-economic context and health care system, expressed in women's, physicians', and men's dispositions (Bourdieu 1977).

In addition to being historically determined, unwanted pregnancies and the spread of STIs were symptoms of severe social dislocation in the aftermath of socialism. Rapid economic stratification and social anomie affected sexual practices and gender relations; new desires and new demands for fulfilling them motivated people to seek out strategies that were not always health-inducing. Disease spread as a result of women's and men's new opportunities to travel abroad and meet people from a variety of backgrounds at home; the proliferation of sexually explicit images in a context where information about sexual health remained marginalized contributed as well. New economic constraints increased the prevalence of prostitution and the informal use of sex for personal profit (Rethman 2001). Unwanted pregnancies and disease were also caused by sexual violence and abuse, issues that remained unexamined by educators and the media alike, except as anomalous acts by deranged strangers (Johnson 2004). Sexual trends in Russia were the outcomes of social and systemic forces, products of the hypocrisies of the Soviet era and those of democratizing "freedoms," no less than individual choices. Incorporating such insights into educational programs could, I thought, raise people's critical consciousness regarding the state's power in their lives and provide an impetus for political engagement in response.

Yet providers failed to capture these complex causes when they lamented the "lack of *kul'turnost'*" and stressed the need for patients to develop their *lichnosti*. When threatening about the dangers of sexual activity and abortion, or even when asserting the "natural" character of sexual pleasure, educators prescribed individualizing types of cures. This conceptual lens predominated, I will show, because it was both suited to widespread understandings about the futility of political engagement and flexible enough to generate multiple, even contradictory, strategies for channeling individual agency.

The promotion of personal work on the self was not something new for Russian professionals. In the decades preceding the Bolshevik Revolution, Russian lawyers and doctors interrogated the causes of social ills by examining individual forms of degeneracy. For example, inspired by European theories of criminal anthropology, many explained prostitution as a sign of innate criminal and sexual deviance among lower class women (Engelstein 1992b). The focus on the individual as potentially antisocial and degenerate became institutionalized in official policies during Stalinism. That regime coerced individual displays of loyalty and conformity, and encouraged people's purposeful self-fashioning as heroic collectivists (Kharkhordin 1999). Medical experts played an important role in these processes during and after Stalinism (Field 1996). Physicians' health education courses focused on disciplining bodily practices to conform to standards of proper hygiene and sexual restraint. Moreover, by making the body an instrument of control, physicians established a normative vision of respectable selfhood [*kul'turnost'*] based on compliance with scientific authority. In the 1990s, many of these familiar discourses continued: physician-educators urged people to channel sexual activity into morally acceptable purposes, and many construed bodily practices as indicators of the quality of people's characters. Soviet historical experience played an important role in the individualizing paths of social change that predominated in sex education. These discourses also gave deprofessionalized medical workers a means of shoring up their social authority under conditions where political-economic influence remained elusive.

But to end the analysis here risks appearing to suggest that post-Soviet health education mechanistically reproduced long-standing patterns of discipline. Although the ongoing ways that deprofessionalization helped make processes of medicalization ideologically attractive for providers were important, it is no less significant that health education courses differed widely in their messages. If all educators agreed on the need for personal moral revivals, they deployed concepts of *kul'turnost'* and *lichnost'* differently, stretching and projecting them to fit larger, often competing visions of change. This chapter compares the educational work of gynecologists and psychologists to highlight such subtleties. Specifically, as gynecologists urged young women to "raise their level of culture" in sexual behavior and personal hygiene, they depicted patient compliance as essential to physical and moral purity. Psychologists, by contrast, experimented with forms of social control emphasizing patients' self-knowledge and emphasized the development of personalities unencumbered by obligations to a larger *kollektiv.* In their view, ignorance and illness, abortions and sexually transmitted infections, were symptoms of psychological defects caused by Soviet policies on censorship and repression; individual moral development for patients *as well as other providers* was considered a means of healing the social scars inflicted by the Soviet system. While retaining essentialist notions of gender, their messages urged women and men to become knowledgeable about their bodies, their pleasures, and their human natures. They constructed professional authority as a source of support helping people move beyond what they perceived as the injurious strictures inherited from Soviet history.

Analyzing these lectures as a feminist anthropologist has proved challenging. On the one hand, my commitment to the critique of medicalization has inclined me to highlight how providers' aversion to collective action for women's health, and their focus on reviving expert authority, maintained women's systemic disempowerment under post-Soviet conditions. On the other hand, the goal of exposing disciplinary practices must remain compatible with ethnographic sensitivity to cultural knowledge, in its local distinctions and shifting forms. For example, whether providers portrayed sex as pathological or pleasurable narrowed or broadened the range of practices sanctioned by professional authority. The investments some providers made in a humanistic, individualized subject offered wider imaginative possibilities than demands for conformity presented by others. Such struggles over the content of health and sex education evident in providers' competing messages had important, pragmatic consequences for women's lives. Thus, while I recognize that health education projects shared the vision of individualizing disciplinary change, I eschew foregone conclusions that *any* move toward emancipation within this rubric was illusory. A view of discourse as power, and education as discipline, need not foreclose recognition of strategic, if limited, emancipatory effects (Lock and Kaufert 1998); indeed, such nuanced attention is necessary for understanding the pragmatic struggles and incremental achievements of everyday life after socialism.

I begin with a brief historical overview of Soviet-era state-sponsored approaches to sexual health (frequently termed "sexual hygiene" [*seksual'naia gigienia*] or "sexual moral education" [*polovoe vospitanie*]), which provided the background for educational work in the 1990s. Drawing on fieldwork in clinics and schools where physicians lectured teenagers on reproductive health, I present the major approaches to cultivating personal moral change that health educators pursued. The first group, consisting mostly of gynecologists, reproduced Soviet approaches of advocating personal hygiene, discipline, and sexual restraint as they confined sexuality to a renewed maternal subjectivity for women. Another group of educators, mainly psychologists, worked to debunk Soviet "myths" and taboos by redefining sexuality and sexual pleasure as "natural" and necessary for a well-developed, individualized personality. Yet even while urging the renewed value of individuality, their discussions implicitly reconfirmed the public struggles for control over sexuality by families and professionals alike.

Educators attempted to protect Russian youth from the perceived dangers associated with the breakdown of the socialist regime. Here one could imagine educators embracing a politicized message highlighting the loss of health care and other social rights and inspiring public organizing as a path for social change. Instead, however, educators fought against the collapse of social control by targeting individual sexual behaviors alone. But again, different professionals pursued this task differently. Gynecologists portrayed sexually active youth as spiritually lost, diseased, and depraved through moral dissolution. They urged compliance with expert knowledge by threatening that disobedience would bring physical pollution and social exclusion, thus blaming ill and marginalized populations for their plight. In contrast, psychologists strove to acknowledge the complex emotions surrounding sexuality instead of blaming individuals who engaged in risky behavior. They warned of the "cruelties" one may encounter "out there" in society, and offered practical steps for recognizing and coping with social dangers. Psychologist-educators recognized that the legitimacy of medical power had been deeply shaken by ideological and structural forces associated with Soviet officialdom. As they sought to revive professional authority in their lectures, they did so not through threats about the price of disobedience, but through establishing medical power as *benevolent,* and distinct from the larger state system. All these experts, explicitly or implicitly, conceptualized the state and society as dangerous, ill-inducing forces, and they located the necessary tactics for health and safety in a newly developed and disciplined self. But their practices of inspiring moral change, and the expressions of individual subjectivity they deemed acceptable, diverged profoundly.

HISTORICIZING SEXUAL DISCIPLINE

"Moral education" [*polovoe vospitanie*] was a genre of education created under Stalin and expounded throughout the Soviet era. It involved teaching and modeling the behaviors consistent with a "proper upbringing," captured in the notion of "culturedness" [*kul'turnost'*]. To advance "culturedness" among the population, state bureaucrats and medical experts in the 1920s launched a massive attack on disorder, dirt, and indecency—portrayed as interchangeable categories[3]—in favor of order and hygiene as the paths to health and moral purity. These qualities came to symbolize the basic requisites for the "high level of culture" associated with a "civilized," urban life under modernity (Volkov 2000). They were advocated incessantly in the state's universalizing, disciplining projects for moral education, *vospitanie,* which became the exclusive form of knowledge transmission in health education texts for popular consumption.

Sexuality per se became publicly addressed—even indirectly—only with Khrushchev's new policies, which aimed to relax state surveillance and open up society. However, the state's attitude toward sexuality and reproduction during this period of "the thaw" continued to associate individual and national health with "moral purity," defined as sexual restraint. Women's nature was maternal, and the imperative of reproduction informed all sexually related discussions. To protect their fertility, moreover, women needed to follow the rules of hygiene. It was under the rubric of "hygiene" that processes of menstruation and conception were described; texts generally included no details of sexual intercourse. The tone was didactic, with physicians appropriating the right to control individual sexual behavior in the name of society's interests. A sex education manual from 1958 exemplifies this tendency:

> It is generally known that the behavior of a person in questions of love, marriage, and family, the correct and sensible organization of his personal life, have a great influence on productive and societal work, on all creative activities of the person . . . and on the life of all society as a whole. That is why sexual relations of people are not the personal affair of each separate person, but the affair of all of society. (A.G. Stankov, *Polovaia zhizin' v sem'ia* 1958, cited in Field 1996: 129)[4]

A main aspect of "society's interest" in sexuality involved ensuring the continuous, successful reproduction of the Soviet population in politically desirable quantities. Stalin had tried to affect this process by criminalizing abortion, but the numerous deaths and complications resulting from underground abortions proved the futility of prohibition. To prevent such widespread, detrimental health effects, Khrushchev decriminalized abortion in 1955. Far from establishing a woman's rights to autonomy and individual decision-making over her body, however, legalization was intended as the first step toward eradication of abortion (Goldman 1993). Consequently, newly published texts on "sexual hygiene" in the 1950s and 60s presented an overtly negative stance toward abortion. In their clinical practice and "enlightenment work" (mandatory community public health service) gynecologists were instructed to struggle actively against women's use of the procedure while promoting marriage and motherhood as alternatives (Field 1996: 15). Contraceptives were difficult to obtain and quite often not used at all (Remennick 1991, 1993).

Anti-abortion literature portrayed abortion as a "betrayal of women's maternal nature," reasoning that with the generous maternity benefits offered by the Soviet state, women had no reason not to have large families. Those who sought abortions were characterized as selfish and frivolous, motivated by the desire to "enjoy themselves" rather than to fulfill their maternal nature. Women were warned that aborting the first pregnancy could cause them to become infertile, a status that would threaten their marriage and put their womanhood into doubt. Pamphlets often depicted women suffering from deep regret after terminating a pregnancy, but blamed them for having brought "the agony of unfulfilled maternal feelings" on themselves (Field 1996). Notably, abortion was not defined as "murder," since communism's materialism and atheism determined that personhood began only at birth. Rather, abortion was seen as a highly risky act: with ruinous consequences for one's reproductive health, it represented both physical danger and social pollution.

Sex education literature also deemed it necessary for young men to achieve moral purity. In their case, however, the challenge involved actively suppressing sexual desire, portrayed as a ubiquitous but ultimately resolvable problem. It was the "problem" of masturbation that information pamphlets for the sexual moral education of young men addressed. Masturbation was portrayed as siphoning off energy from important productive labor and leading young men to be apathetic, pessimistic, and individualistic—antisocial characteristics that a communist society would not tolerate (Field 1996: 18–20). Through inner strength and will power, young men—like adult men who have mastered the demands of a "cultured" life—were told to switch their attention away from sexual urges and toward the collective.

THE "DEMOGRAPHIC CRISIS": REVISING SEXUAL MORAL EDUCATION TO PROMOTE LARGER, HAPPIER FAMILIES

In the early 1970s, demographers announced that below-replacement fertility rates in European regions of the USSR amounted to an urgent "demographic crisis" (Lapidus 1978; Attwood 1990). Small families and high divorce rates were interpreted by these scientists, educators, and policymakers to reflect a breakdown in the value of family life, attributed largely to women's participation in the labor force. Early socialist ideals concerning the need for gender equality were now viewed as misguided, and the policies that resulted from the concept of women's "emancipation" were blamed for having brought the nation to the brink of catastrophe: with no change in fertility rates over the next decades, demographers warned, the Russian nation would begin to die out.

Following the announcement of the "demographic crisis," several important changes occurred in moral education about sexuality. By the mid 1980s, instead of focusing on the suppression of sexuality and eradication of masturbation, discourses assumed a new emphasis—strengthening individual desires for family life. This goal was to be accomplished through pedagogical campaigns intended to cultivate femininity and masculinity and improve the "culture" of male-female interactions. Specifically, demographers and pedagogues devised pro-natalist "sex-role socialization" classes, and in 1984, a course on "Ethics and Psychology of Family Life" became compulsory for ninth- and tenth-graders. The explicit objectives of this course were that young citizens would embrace rigid visions of proper sex roles and would aspire to have three or more children as both a social obligation and personal desire (Attwood 1990).[5] *Kul'turnost'*, or culturedness, continued to be invoked as a scheme for proper behavior and etiquette in personal interactions, while women and men were now instructed that being a cultured, moral person required them to realize the dictates of their gendered "nature." While in Western Europe and North America the women's movement seized upon images of sexual equality and egalitarian relations between men and women became increasingly popular, Soviet experts claimed the need to "raise the culture of male-female interactions" by modifying girls' and women's behavior. Sexual moral education texts, including the textbook for the "Ethics and Psychology of Family Life" course, elaborated vivid attacks on "emancipated" (used pejoratively to mean autonomous, ambitious, assertive) women.

Notably, the demographic crisis also brought about a gradual reconsideration of sexual practices, including masturbation. With the state's priority clearly focused on the promotion of stable and fertile families, deterring boys from masturbation became less important and was seen as possibly more harmful than useful. Demographers' and educators' concern to ensure a "successful" family life that would lead to increased fertility prompted attention to problems of impotence and sexual frustration. Specifically, texts elaborated a new approach to masturbation that was intended to minimize the consequences resulting from the public anxiety focused on the practice. One manual on sexual moral education written for parents and published in 1982 emphasized that masturbation was a "physically harmless" practice if performed "in moderation." The text warned parents and teachers that *their* negative attitudes toward masturbation lead boys to suffer neuroses, psychologically induced impotence, and a catastrophic future family life (Khipkovoi, Vul'fov, and Grebennikov 1982: 63–65). While as late as 1990 masturbation was still associated with social problems and "spiritual illness," (Loseva 1990: 13), parents were cautiously instructed not to denounce the practice but to distract their sons from masturbating by encouraging their involvement in other activities, such as sports (Khipkovoi, Vul'fov, and Grebennikov 1982: 65–66). What is notably absent from these texts is any reference to girls and masturbation. In this 1982 text, for example, the issue of masturbation was placed under the section "A Boy Becomes a Young Man"; in the companion section, "A Girl Becomes a Young Woman," however, the discussion was limited to menstruation, the development of breasts, and the importance of proper hygiene. I have found no direct association between women and sexual desire or pleasure until the post-Soviet era.

Moreover, texts on sexual moral education devoted minimal attention to birth control methods. From the early 1970s on, the Soviet Ministry of Health expressed doubts about the safety of oral contraceptives, disparagingly referring to them as "hormones." While the strong doses of early generations of the pill were blamed for causing excessive hair growth, weight gain, and nausea, no research was done to modify the pill and ameliorate these side effects—it was merely withdrawn from most state distribution networks. Until quite recently medical experts and laypersons alike have considered the pill more dangerous than abortions. Nor were condoms widely imported, and those that were domestically produced were perceived to be of poor quality. Nonetheless, in estimates of contraceptive use from the 1980s, condoms and IUDs were the most popular methods, used by 9–25 percent of respondents (Remennick 1993; Visser, Bruyniks, and Remennick 1993). Given the relatively low use of contraceptives and widespread reliance on abortion to control fertility, it is notable that texts on sexual health and sexual moral education were typically vague about contraceptive methods. To the extent that birth control was mentioned, it was portrayed as the province of physicians—experts whose esoteric knowledge made them alone capable of determining the appropriate methods for women.

The public discipline of intimate behavior was the overriding purpose of publications concerning sexual and reproductive health. Texts focused on the need to correct women who raised their daughters to loathe or infantilize men and/or spurn sex (Loseva 1990: 30). Blaming emasculating, aggressive wives for high divorce rates, moral sex education discourses held women responsible or blameworthy in practically every account of social and familial problems. Typical manuals on sex education in the 1980s and early 1990s retained didactic instruction in the behaviors and attitudes necessary for a stable and happy family. Authors frequently claimed that citizens are obligated to assume responsibility for resolving the demographic crisis by realizing the collective and personal need for more children (e.g., Loseva 1990: 26–27).

DEFINING PLEASURE AND DANGER FOR A POST-SOVIET CONSCIOUSNESS

Since the late 1980s, Russian society has considered itself in the midst of a "sexual revolution." In large part, this sensation was a response to the abrupt introduction of sexually explicit media and publications that ensued with glasnost. When television and newspapers first began to detail such phenomena as prostitution, group sex, rape, and child abuse, waves of shock, confusion, and titillation swept a society unaccustomed to any public discussion of sexual matters. (Kon 1995: 103). The media, reveling in the demise of prohibition, found its voice in sensationalism. Sexually explicit language and erotic scenes quickly became commonplace on prime time television, and for the first time ever pornography became readily available if not practically ubiquitous in streetside kiosks. The eminent Russian sociologist Igor Kon describes the public's response to this media carnival, in which sexual frankness came to stand for broader political questions, such as the moral status of democratic change:

> Sexual symbols and values, which earlier had been peripheral to the ideological nucleus of culture, now became a sort of watershed dividing "right" and "left," as well as the generations. Sexuality quickly began to polarize and politicize. This created a host of very acute political, moral, and aesthetic problems that society was just as ill-equipped to understand—let alone resolve—as had been the universally damned state power. (Kon 1995: 101–2)

As in most countries around the world, the need for providing sex education to schoolchildren and teenagers in Russia has been far from universally accepted.[6] As Kon indicates, many in the older generation, along with those opposed to the democratization of the political system and liberalization of society more generally, expressed outright disdain for sex education initiatives. Moreover, as data about fertility decline mounted, conservative and nationalist organizations opposing it gained political strength by portraying sex education as a foreign-sponsored effort to hasten the demise of the nation by teaching Russian children "to reject childbearing" (Bateneva 1997; Medvedeva and Shishova 2000). Projects for sex education and family planning became maligned as channels for importing "Western cultural evils"—including homosexuality and depopulation (Kon 1997: 399–400)—and many were cancelled. In these campaigns nationalists were supported by the Orthodox Church, which argued that the loss of social and spiritual order required a return to Orthodox morality and the "national moral-ethical conceptions and traditions of the peoples of Russia" (Kon 1997: 404). In 1997, conservative legislators, responding to the public's and the Church's outcry over pornography and population decline, withdrew funding for the newly created Russian Family Planning Association, while stressing the need to protect Russian traditions and values from the onslaught of a "Western" takeover. Such campaigns were ironic, given that Russian family planning programs and sex education work have not promoted Western notions of "choice" and "freedom," but rather stressed the need for reviving moral purity, strengthening families, and containing sexuality within the bounds of marriage (Rivkin-Fish 1999, in press).

Poised in this hostile context, gynecologists and psychotherapists conducting sex education were a uniquely motivated group. In our conversations, they framed their mission with enthusiasm and urgency, and viewed their work as a calling.[7] They used the public hospitals and outpatient clinics where they worked as a base; until the late 1990s, sex educators also conducted outreach at neighborhood schools, whose administrators looked to physicians to provide authoritative knowledge on sexuality. With no set curriculum or official guidelines (and no budget for supplies), educators created patchworks of material gathered from personal libraries and donated by Western humanitarian organizations, missionaries, and commercial firms. In some cases, they welcomed assistance offered by international anti-abortion organizations such as Focus on the Family and Human Life International, whose messages of family values and spiritual renewal after communism helped local educators assert the legitimacy of their work. These organizations also provided extensive resources for some local women's health clinics, repairing their decrepit infrastructures and supplying updated, comfortable furniture, video machines, and abundant literature and films on the harms of abortion—such as *The Silent Scream.* Other institutions worked with a range of international organizations, including WHO and family planning associations. Working with teenagers was a priority.[8]

Though lectures spanned a range of topics, only a minimal amount of time was devoted to descriptions of physiological processes surrounding puberty, menstruation, and conception. Indeed, to the extent that these topics were addressed, they often remained framed as issues of "hygiene."

A lecture series at a St. Petersburg teen center for reproductive health, for example, included "The Physiological Specificities of the Puberty Period and Foundations of a Healthy Life Style," "Care for the Skin and Hair," and a lecture sponsored by a tampon company, titled "Personal Hygiene for Teenagers, A Deposit for Your Success—Tambrands, St. Petersburg." Free samples of Tampax tampons and educational brochures in Russian were distributed to the audience. Most lectures, however, concentrated explicitly on conveying moral concerns about sexuality and reproduction, including "Sex before 18: Health, Spirituality [*dukhovnost'*], Beauty"; other themes mentioned included the difference between sex and love and the importance of romance and spirituality in relationships. As public criticism mounted throughout the 1990s that sex education threatened the nation's vitality by encouraging contraception and lowering the birth rate, physician-educators' focus on strengthening families and individual morality became an important means of defending their work.

GYNECOLOGISTS AND THE PROMOTION OF MATERNAL RESPONSIBILITY

Much of the thirteen lectures I attended and taped in 1994–95 reproduced to a greater or lesser extent Soviet-era discourses on *polovoe vospitanie,* or sexual moral education. For example, some educators emphasized the need to promote disciplined "hygiene" behavior in young women, encouraging them to view and care for their bodies as a vessel whose main purpose was to reproduce. This was evident in the lecture of one obstetrician in her late thirties, whose audience consisted of about ten girls aged nine to eleven. Nadezhda Nikolaevna described motherhood as the central goal of the female reproductive system, even to the point of scientific inaccuracy. Pointing to a drawing of female anatomy, she explained:

> Here, near the uterus is the ovary. This is your most important organ when you will be women. It is here in the ovary that you have the egg cell, out of which later will come a child. None of you have gotten your period yet, but in your ovaries all your future eggs are already there. That is, in your ovaries are all the egg cells, which are, so to speak, sitting and waiting for their time. And for each of these egg cells will come a moment when it will mature, get up *and be fertilized.* [*I dlia kazhdoi etoi iaitsekletki pridet moment, kogda imenno ona sozreet, podnimetsia i budet oplodotvorena*].

The erroneous assertion that *each egg* will be fertilized is telling for more than the fact that it was a mistake. Even if we assume that Nadezhda Nikolaevna meant to say that each egg has a chance to be fertilized, her statement achieved the sense of an imperative—the female body will conceive and bear children, and that is virtually the only thing it can and should do. She defined the egg cell as the entity "out of which later will come a child," and further depicted it as "waiting for its time" to be fertilized.

She did not describe the process of conception itself, or explain that menstrual cycles are the outcomes of eggs that have not been fertilized. (Following her lecture, she showed a foreign-made cartoon with Russian voice-overs that explained these processes.) But her discussion offered a striking discussion of women's motherhood without mentioning men, sex, or sperm at all—as if the egg spontaneously and autonomously transformed into a fetus. While Soviet-era texts usually did include discussion of male sex cells, they too remained vague on the question of how the sperm cells actually made their way to the egg.

After presenting the female body as a budding source of maternity, Nadezhda Nikolaevna then emphasized the need for the girls to develop the proper habits of cleanliness and bodily surveillance and the readiness to submit to expert authority in the case of anomaly, to ensure that their reproductive capacity would be uninhibited. Implicit in this conceptual approach to the female body lurked the ever-present danger of infertility:

> Here's what you need to know now: you will all soon begin your periods. For some of you it will come this year, for some it will come next year, and for some it will begin at age fourteen. How should you behave yourself? [*Kak nado vesti sebia?*] Girls, please remember, that if suddenly you get an inflammation of the uterus or [tape unclear], that can result in infertility. . . .
>
> Remember this, please. When your period begins, it is important to take care of yourself very carefully [*sledit' za soboi osobenno vnimatel'no*], because . . . that is, now you should wash yourselves not twice a day as usual, but as much as possible [*kak mozhno chashche*]. If there's an opportunity to go and wash yourself, it's necessary to do so, necessary to change your pad.

She went on to tell girls to record the dates and lengths of their periods on a calendar, and always to refer to the calendar when arriving for a gynecological exam. "In case your period is inconsistent, it comes early or late, you'll know through your calendar that the cycle has broken down." Asserting the need for girls to record their cycles, and immediately report any breakdowns or "inflammations" to the gynecologist who would then intervene to ensure no threats existed to their fertility, Nadezhda Nikolaevna worked to create a new generation of patients compliant with medical power and authority.

Another tactic deployed from Soviet education was the "discourse of blame" that Humphrey (1983) first identified and that Field (1996) found prevailing in literature on abortion since the mid 1950s. One fieldwork experience in 1993 demonstrated this approach most vividly. In the waiting area of a women's clinic in St. Petersburg, I saw color photographs of aborted fetuses lining the walls. When I asked the deputy director of the clinic why this material was placed in the site where women sat before receiving abortions, she responded matter-of-factly, saying: "We hope to discourage women from having abortions" (Rivkin-Fish 1994).

I soon learned that this approach was far from unusual among Russian educators. Anastasia Pavlovna was a gynecologist in her mid forties who was active in sex education programs at her clinic. Her strategies deployed blame and guilt tactics, and also incorporated new concepts garnered from her exposure to the global anti-abortion movement. Unlike Soviet-era anti-abortion messages, for example, she described the fetus as an individual [*lichnost'*] and defined abortion as "murder." Speaking to a group of young women at the teenage center, she gave her audience "information" about the clinic's abortion services, while warning them about what the procedure "actually" entails:

> You must know this: We do abortions up to twelve weeks of pregnancy. The little child [*rebenochek*] is already pretty big. . . . At twelve weeks everything is already visible on the [ultrasound] film: the head, fingers, little hands, little feet. But I tell the girl (having an ultrasound before getting an abortion): "I won't show you." Because he's like a prisoner in solitary confinement waiting for the death sentence to be carried out.

Without explicitly commenting on her efforts to transcend Soviet ideology, Anastasia Pavlovna used language that markedly opposed Soviet materialism and atheism. She attributed personhood to the fetus and asserted that by the fifth month, abortion is "a sin against God." Long-standing discourses of blame were refined to warn women that not only abortions but even undesired pregnancies have consequences on another individual's [*lichnost'*] life. "Babies" in utero suffer if they are unwanted, she insisted, "I want you to remember: that baby—it already understands if it's needed, if it was conceived by love or by chance, if nobody needs it, neither its father nor its mother. . . . This child's . . . entire short life is full of suffering, pain, tears which its mother doesn't hear."

Anastasia Pavlovna and others argued against abortion (and implicitly against Soviet ideology) by constructing the fetus as a conscious, individual being with emotions and the ability to suffer. Connected to this was the familiar notion that women who abort were alienated from their maternal natures and lacked a moral understanding of how to live in a "cultured" way. Women needed to know that motherhood was the expected outcome of sexual activity; educators admonished their teenage listeners to be mindful of this moral burden when making their decisions about whether or not to become sexually active. In messages that reproduced long-standing concerns for promoting discipline, responsibility, and *kul'-turnost'*, these educational strategies targeted individual behavior through guilt, blame, and moral absolutes.

Despite their strident opposition to abortion, these educators tended to provide few details about the range of contraceptive methods and specific ways to utilize them; I heard no information about their various risks and estimated degrees of reliability. Though mentioned sporadically and often interspersed with other topics, birth control was frequently associated with insecure and impoverished relationships. Again, I quote from Anastasia Pavlovna: "There are girls [who say,] 'Oh, I don't know what to do with him. I love him very much, but he's not loyal.' I can't tell them, 'How can you let this go on!' That's useless. So I'll say to them, 'If you can't avoid it in any way, and your heart and your head are at odds, then use a condom.' It's the only method of protection against STIs and pregnancy."

In this comment, birth control was constructed as necessary in unfortunate cases where the irrational pangs of love and desire reign over one's better logic. Implicitly, the condom became a sign that protection is needed because a given relationship lacks the expected criteria of loyalty and decency.[9] She portrayed relationships where birth control is a central variable as unfortunate and rather degraded in their failure to become a steppingstone to marriage and family. The idea that pregnancies could or should be "planned" was not incorporated into the efforts to reduce the use of abortion. In discourses that echoed "family hygiene" lectures of the 1960s, sex was depicted as a step toward motherhood, and motherhood or abortion were portrayed as the inevitable outcomes of sexual activity.[10] For both Nadezhda Nikolaevna and Anastasia Pavlovna, the goal of health education was to promote personal discipline in caring for the body as a vehicle of maternity. Learning to behave as a responsible future mother required hygienic skills and habits for cleanliness as well as a nonfrivolous attitude toward sexuality as a direct step toward parenthood. Those who failed to comply with these imperatives were to blame for their problems.

PSYCHOLOGISTS AND THE DEVELOPMENT OF INDIVIDUAL CHARACTER

Paulina Aleksandrovna, a psychotherapist in her mid thirties, approached the problem of abortion in a strikingly different way. When I first met her in 1995, she was developing sex education in schools and working as the president of an anti-abortion movement in St. Petersburg. She explained abortion practices as a widespread effect of failed interpersonal communication and domestic conflicts, which ultimately, she believed, stemmed from inadequate state policies:

Why do women get abortions? If we talk about it on one level, OK, we can say there's a low level of sexual culture. We don't manage much with contraceptives, and there's no sex education. In the family, the parents don't talk about it, nor do they in schools. But it's more than that. It's about the interrelations between husband and wife, about their responsibility to each other. They don't understand each other.

This lack of understanding was expressed through mutual blame, anger, and aggression, conflictual interactions. Often the failures and anxiety were linked to unrealized images of masculinity and femininity and to unfulfilled expectations of gender roles and responsibilities. Her explanation relied on an image of women and men shaped by unchanging natural differences that could be traced to prehistoric times—when men hunted and brought back food, and women cared for children and preserved the hearth. Modern societies, the Soviet Union among them, had strained these natural roles by subverting its traditional division of labor. As a result of this, women and men suffered from feelings of inadequacy and distress, and a disturbed imbalance in interpersonal relations:

> As a psychoanalyst, I see the women I work with—why do they get abortions? [A woman says of her husband:] "He's not capable of doing anything! There are no men!" . . . [So she says to her husband], "I had an abortion, now give me money. You didn't bring . . . me meat, and I have nothing to protect. I'm not a woman." And modern women don't know how to be women, and men are afraid of this. Women need to preserve themselves, their feminine source . . . the instinct to give birth.

In this view, marital disharmony, abortions, and low "sexual culture" all derived from a painful loss of traditional gender roles. Men "aren't capable" of providing for their families; women "don't know how" to be feminine, maternal. Abortions signaled the inability of men and women to nurture their families and care for each other. Yet if Paulina Aleksandrovna located the problems in interpersonal relations, she traced the roots of these ills to the state's inability to enable women and men to fulfill their "natural" functions:

> Here in the twentieth century, we're having a big crisis; there's a lot of uncertainty about male-female relations. We don't know what a woman's role in society should be. We say we can't give birth to many children because we don't have enough money, we have great financial problems. Yet in the U.S. and Europe, people have a car, a home, but no child. We [in Russia] have a patriarchal, traditional country. For women, this patriarchal system assigns her only the role of housewife, and she doesn't want that. All over the world, governmental systems don't give women the opportunity to both take care of their family and develop themselves in society. Women can't fulfill both roles. This is the tragedy we're dealing with.

While this comment appeared to acknowledge the need for politically based efforts to improve women's health, Paulina Aleksandrovna rejected the idea that pursuing a state-based solution through advocacy of specific legislation or public policies was the answer. I suggested that if governments failed to address women's needs, perhaps we should encourage women to become more active in leading the country and addressing women's concerns. Her answer came swiftly and without a trace of ambivalence: "No, a woman who goes into government won't be able to remain a woman. She must behave as the system requires, she'll be forced to. What we need is something different. If women went into government, this would take them away from the family. . . . When women go into the government, they go in as men."

Because abortion was a symptom of the widespread impoverishment of family relations and the lack of mutual love and understanding between spouses, as well as the consequence of lax moral education [*vospitanie*], what was needed, she argued, was an all-out effort to morally educate women and men, to develop their sense of "self," and to allow them to fulfill their gender-based "functions" or natures. "We need to focus on the harmony in the family, on interrelations," she explained.

Sensitive to the complex challenges women confront as they deal with their husbands and jobs, their sense of identity, and their severe economic constraints, Paulina Aleksandrovna did not blame women for having abortions. Nor did she find politics a productive approach to reducing abortions. In 1995, Paulina Aleksandrovna expressed ambivalence about the political dimension of anti-abortion work and rejected the idea of criminalization. Even while serving as a leader of Right to Live, she told me she tried to avoid the "political work." She put her faith in the process of moral education [*vospitanie*], to help young adults develop the emotional awareness and strength needed to forge emotionally sound interpersonal relations and families:

> Abortion is immoral, it is murder. But how to go about dealing with it as an ethical problem is very difficult. . . . The problem is that in our conditions today, I can't tell a woman, "You're killing your baby." It's very difficult, we have to bring people to the point that morally, they understand it. As you can't bring someone to that moral level by making it illegal, that doesn't work. . . . The moral development of personalities [*vospitanie lichnosti*] begins even before conception. So it's very important to prepare people to be parents, to morally educate [*vospitivat*] them. . . . It's a question of how the father and mother relate to each other. We need to educate them.

In 2000, I met Paulina Aleksandrovna again and learned she had quit working with Right to Live, which subsequently folded in St. Petersburg. She focused her energies on helping teens find meaning in their lives and offering social support, rather than what she described as the more narrow, political issue of fighting abortion.

DEBUNKING SOVIET MYTHS, TRANSCENDING THE SOVIET ORDER

Igor Mikhailovich, a psychotherapist, and Yuri Grigorovich, an obstetrician with psychotherapeutic training, also had different agendas for cultivating moral personhood. They viewed Soviet ideology as a source of blatant falsehoods, dangerous myths, and repressive taboos that distorted Russians' notions of sexuality and ruined their sexual experience. In their lectures and interviews, they remarked on the widespread ignorance about sexual anatomy that plagued Russian society and led to breakdowns in intimate relations, unfulfilled marriages, and individual anxieties and traumas. For example, Igor Mikhailovich told of phone calls received on the clinic's anonymous hotline from teenage girls asking how to insert tampons and stressed the importance for young people to know and understand their bodies. The focus of their lectures was the need to debunk Soviet-era myths regarding sexuality, sexual pleasure, and "alternative" forms of sexual experience, such as masturbation. One lecture in the spring of 1995 took place in a large classroom of a St. Petersburg high school. The principal of the school invited Yuri Grigorovich to give a two-hour lecture on all realms of sexuality education. Over fifty high school boys aged fourteen to seventeen sat in desks arranged in two long rows that spanned the length of the classroom. Yuri Grigorovich began his talk with a fervent insistence that earlier Soviet attempts to repress or rid society of sex were wrong. Sex is not only "normal," he declared, but "important" and "natural." Speaking to his raucous audience with a firm sense of authority, he asserted:

> You know teachers who are afraid—well, speaking honesty, they're afraid to tell you anything, [to deal with] any issues at all associated with the interrelations between the sexes. Well, I want to tell you, my friends, that sexuality is an inseparable part of human existence. And no matter what they have or haven't told you, sexuality is just as much a part of human existence as drinking, breathing, etc. And therefore, to speak of sexuality as something sinful is fairly unjust, and, I would say, even pathological.

Following this statement, he devoted extensive attention to normalizing one of the main practices Soviet ideology had demonized—masturbation:

> Please remember, contemporary sexology views masturbation as an absolutely nor-

mal phenomenon on the path to psychosexual development as a teenager, young man, and adult man. Moreover . . . I want to say immediately, that masturbation, onanism, at present is also viewed as a substitute form, a so-called alternative to the sex act. . . . And in order to take all the humor out of it completely, I want to tell you that 97 percent of teenagers masturbate before beginning a regular sex life.

The rehabilitation of masturbation as a "normal" and "natural" practice was a common objective of lectures conducted by psychotherapists. Committed to a renewed societal interest in the individual, they sought to legitimize nonprocreative (heterosexual) sex, undertaken for pleasure alone. Speaking with a group of ten or so teenage girls in the teenage reproductive center's auditorium, psychotherapist Igor Mikhailovich emphasized the importance for women to be informed about their anatomy, erotic zones, and the "natural" character of sexual pleasure. Firmly committed to instilling in young women and men a sense of the "naturalness" and "necessity" sexuality, he also portrayed himself in explicit opposition to the ideology of the Soviet regime: "If I had given this lecture during the Soviet era, I'd have been sentenced for eight to ten years for the crime of 'perverting a minor.' But now, thankfully, times have changed. . . . No matter how blasphemous it sounds, I recommend this very intimate thing —although each to her own—in principle, a woman must caress herself."

With a substantial dose of sarcasm, he opposed the content of his lectures to "the taboos" constructed by "our wonderful Soviet regime," explaining that the silence long surrounding sexuality had been harmful and inappropriate. Moreover, he forcefully argued that, in contrast to the claims of Soviet ideology, sex is not a perversion, and that minors—children, even babies—are sexual beings. Teaching women that sexual pleasure was important and that it required knowing about their bodies were among his central concerns. His lectures prescribed the cultivation of self-knowledge through specific habits of caring for the self. For example, he painted his audience of young women a scene to help them imagine how they might cultivate this sense of an individual self:

Stay home alone, so nobody will see you or disturb you. Light some candles, put on music—not technopop that gets your neck out of joint—but Mozart, Vivaldi, Bach, and get into the atmosphere. Put on your best dress, stand in front of a large mirror, look at yourself and tell yourself, "I'm beautiful, I'm unique and irreplaceable." . . . Consider yourself a creation of divine significance.

In advocating masturbation as a means for women to learn about their sexual nature and appreciate the uniqueness of the self, he defined individual sexuality as a subject for health: equating healthy sexuality with a healthy self, he taught that women should be familiar with their anatomy;

through knowing their body, women can learn to enjoy and appreciate their physical and spiritual uniqueness. To attain this individual form of sexual health, a woman should engage in individualized practices, spend time alone, get dressed up, listen to music, emotionally take care of herself. With the right approach and preparation, he implied, caressing one's own body leads to self-knowledge. Healthy sexuality was about a healthy, knowledgeable, individualized self-consciousness.

Neither of these educators felt it sufficient to promote individual needs alone. They argued that for both men and women to enjoy sexual pleasure, it was essential for them to have a firm sense of moral obligations to their partner. Yuri Grigorovich's lectures merged the themes of kul'turnost' and lichnost' to instill in boys a sense of moral obligation toward girls, women, and their future wives. He emphasized that men needed to understand and care for their partner's feelings and needs in sexuality. In the following comment to a group of teenaged boys, he confirmed traditional concepts of male-female differences while trying to cultivate the boys' cultured [kul'turnyi] approach to their girlfriends and future wives:

> It is necessary to know your partner; when there is no knowledge of your partner's body, when the man's goal is to undertake the sex act in order to satisfy himself, the end result is that the partner will either put up with him her whole life, quietly hating [him], or will simply leave him. Knowledge of your partner's body is absolutely necessary not only for a normal sex life but as a consequence, a normal family life. . . . While for the man there's a precise organization of life—career, work, periodic sex acts generally for self-satisfaction—for women the main thing is the family. . . . Please remember that if a girl has sex with you then therefore somewhere in the depths of her soul she sees you as a potential future husband. Think about your responsibility—this person who you supposedly love at the moment, you are basically cruelly deceiving.

Though men found rather easy physical pleasure in "periodic sex acts," Yuri Grigorovich warned, neglect of their partner's pleasure could ruin their marriage. Here, men's recognition of women's emotional and physical needs, a respect of gender differences, was deemed necessary for healthy, mutually respectful marital relations. Caring about women's enjoyment was necessary for a man to be a responsible, decent person.

Igor Mikhailovich similarly qualified the notion that sexuality was "normal," by striving to establish that healthy sexuality required interpersonal care and concern. While depicting the possibilities of sexual expression, he also worked to cultivate people's sense of obligation to each other:

> Any form of interaction with any parts of the body—hands, legs, body, lips, tongue, anything that you want is allowed, which does not entail coercion against another

person, which is between loving people, not moral force, not dependency, or of course physical force. And then with these relations with a beloved person you can reach the peak of sexual satisfaction—orgasm.

For these educators, care for the self and an obligation to ensure individual sexual pleasure and the desires of one's partner provided an explicit means of transcending Soviet-era demands for collectivist concerns that had marginalized and delegitimized sexuality. The cultivation of new attitudes and behaviors around sexual intimacy and self-knowledge became an important means of reviving society through individualizing moral change. Their lectures effected a separation from Soviet ideological "taboos," replacing its prescriptions not with "bare facts" but with a morality of individual selfhood based in interpersonal responsibility and *kul'turnost'*.

PREVENTING DISEASE THROUGH MORAL PERSONHOOD

If Soviet-era "sexophobia" constituted a major source of societal ills in the views of some health educators, all providers whom I spoke with considered post-Soviet public discourses on sexuality to present a new and distinctly menacing set of dangers. Health experts, like many educated Russians in the mid 1990s, lamented the perceived "anything goes" approach of the market-based mass media—the sexually explicit films shown on prime time television, the talk shows obsessively detailing all possible forms of sex, and the plethora of pornographic literature available on almost every street corner of the city. The threats posed by such explosive public discourse were said to be both physical—the rampant spread of sexually transmitted infections, with their attendant consequences of infertility, illness, and even death—and moral, involving the degradation of individuals, families, and, ultimately, the nation. Faced with the sense that an urgent campaign was needed to reinstill moral boundaries against a market society run amok, health educators saw their task as building up the personal moral characters of young adults. What is interesting to note is that the critique of "free speech" or market reforms was not made explicit—nobody argued for a return to censorship or addressed the political-economic aspects of reforms. Whatever precise ideas educators had about the reforms of the last decade, these political dimensions remained in the background as educators portrayed Russian society as dissolving in chaos (Ries 1997). For some, such as Anastasia Pavlovna, the chaos was located in persons, those whose moral characters were so deeply depraved that they personified the loss of social control and degradation; others, such as Igor Mikhailovich, identified the dangers within society, but still sought solutions and protections through moral, personal kinds of development.

For gynecologist Anastasia Pavlovna, the lack of *kul'turnost'* and break-down of moral purity were most clearly captured in a single image of dissolution and depravity—that of the prostitute. In discussing the decision to become sexually active, she warned:

> It's important for you to know that in all countries, among all peoples, virginity, morality, and purity have always been honorable. . . . [Referring to her clinical work] I sometimes say to girls, "How many partners have you had?" [The patient answers,] "I don't know." "What do you mean—[have there been] 5, 10, *15*?" And she says, "Well, more than 30." I say, "You know, to be honest it could be called a profession. If you don't want me to call it a profession, then you need to gather your courage and listen well to me, to what I think is necessary."

With these comments, Anastasia Pavlovna urged young women to develop a cultured attitude toward their body and interpersonal relations, which she equated with a feeling of self-worth [*samootsennost'*]. The proper attitude, she argued, would lead to sexual purity, morality, and happiness, but veering off course led to the loss of love, social acceptance, family, and life itself:

> If there's a feeling of self-worth, that I am unique, that the vagina is part of me, the path on which my beloved will be the first to go, and that only he will go in this world and only my child will go through this path, then you will be guaranteed happiness. But if the vagina becomes—as with many girls—forgive me for the rude comparison—literally a courtyard passageway [*prokhodnoi dvor*] where not only drafts pass through but also those STIs, then there will never be contact between you and your child.

Perceiving the dangers facing women who engaged in the chaotic world of sexual exploration to be so great, Anastasia Pavlovna warned girls that they risked losing their future child's love through the contamination of STIs. She reproduced Soviet discourses of blame to promote moral standards of self-discipline and sexual restraint. Her warnings compiled images of pathology and illness to describe women's bodies, as she warned of death through STDs: "Sometimes I tell girls, 'If you're such a fan and sex is a hobby for you, then you must know that you'll get nothing except an entry in the *Guinness Book of World Records*—and the graveyard cross is nearby. Why? Because as a gynecologist working here everyday, I see syphilis in teenagers no less than twice a week.'"[11]

Psychotherapist Igor Mikhailovich also sought to dissuade young women from beginning sex. The dangers he saw facing women were extensive—from STIs and untimely pregnancy to emotional trauma of betrayal and sexual violence. Yet as an experienced psychotherapist unwilling to deploy guilt and blame tactics, he conveyed a broader understanding of the pressures and desires that influence young women. His lectures offered students insights into the emotional conflicts they experienced and strategies they might use to solve them, rather than portraying sexual activity as a girl's chosen path to moral degradation and prostitution. He sought to inform young women about the manipulative tactics men can use:

> Is sex necessary [for you]? This is the question of questions. When kids write me notes and ask "At what age can I begin having sex?" I never [give a specific age]. Everything in its own time. Every person is a *lichnost'*, individual [*individual'nost'*], and decides themselves the moment of becoming sexually active. But you need to ask yourself the question: Do I need this? Why? What for? Am I not under the thumb of my partner? [*Ne idu li ia na povodu u svoego partnera?*] It often happens that a girl and guy meet at a disco, she is seventeen, he is twenty to twenty-one, he already has some experience. And he considers himself Sylvester Stallone; her friends cry out in envy, "Look what you've caught, such a guy, and we poor things are going to be jealous our whole lives." And you think that you've fallen in love.
>
> Very frequently girls'll say, "I love him."
>
> "And how long have you known him?" I ask.
>
> "A month, two months, but I love him so much I'm willing to give myself to him."
>
> "And do you need this?" I ask.
>
> "I don't know."
>
> "Have you read anything about contraception, prevention, on the biological period of fertility? Do you know anything about condoms?"
>
> "Yes, I've heard about something, but I just love him so much."
>
> And often this love ends with the boy saying, "I see how your eyes glow, you love me, right?" And she breathes deeply and says, "I can't live without you" (laughter in auditorium). "Then let's go to bed, to bed, quickly!" Unfortunately, that's it. If you don't have a powerful sense of self [*ia*], then . . . Ask him, "And you, are you already prepared to be a father? We only know each other for two months. And what's going to happen? What's going to become of us?"

Seen in a context where much education remained threatening and punitive, these comments were significant. Igor Mikhailovich offered young women pragmatic suggestions of how to confront boyfriends who pressured them for sex: "Are you prepared to be a father?" he instructed them to ask. Furthermore, his words of caution focused not on the depravity and social ostracism they risked if becoming sexually active, but on the need to be informed about contraception and other modes of protection they could use. His message about whether to begin sexual activity avoided blanket statements, leaving room for individual circumstances and cases. "I do not know what you, as a unique *lichnost'*, need," he seemed to say, "but as an experienced professional, I can give you insights into how to figure it out."

We don't say not to begin sexual relations. . . . It's each person's private business. In America, smart Mary doesn't allow herself unsafe sex. First of all, because she knows that she's not mature enough materially. Even though she is twenty-four to twenty-five years old, she still didn't finish her education, she didn't save up enough money for life with a child, she doesn't have her own place, her own house. And an abortion will cost her tens of thousands of dollars. So she does petting, and experiences all feelings with a condom, and she is happy, has happy sex, which I wish for you.

Through this image of an American woman who practiced safe sex until "financially ready" to start a family, Igor Mikhailovich suggested that a new form of personal discipline in sexuality was necessary for coping with the constraints of market reforms. The "dangers" in his view were not just sexually transmitted diseases, but individuals' lack of preparation for successfully managing their lives in a market economy.

Igor Mikhailovich stressed that sex must be safe and, unlike many of his colleagues, discussed condom use as a positive form of disease and pregnancy prevention. His message contained practical advice for protecting oneself—not only physically, but also socially—from attacks of sexual promiscuity. He told his audience of teenage girls:

Dangerous sex should be avoided at all times. Catching venereal diseases, especially in causal encounters, in the bed after the disco or having a good time out in nature, at the beach [where there's] music, feelings, a boy, everything is wonderful. Girls must protect themselves, a woman must love her genitals, value her vagina as her overall health. That will be the source of her prosperity.

Use a condom please. Take it out of your purse. I recommend girls carry condoms in their purses, no matter how strange it sounds, always, always. And if a wise mom who sometimes likes to go through her daughter's purse to look at her notes, sees it and faints from shock, [saying,] "What are you doing, can this be *my daughter*? I raised you, I never told you a word that such things happen, and you are allowing yourself this!" You tell her, "Igor Mikhailovich taught me and said that I should do this. Just in case, mom. Everything happens in life. You didn't expect me to be smart this way."

Nonetheless, Igor Mikhailovich did not have sanguine images about the kinds of sexual experience most teenagers have. The world outside the safe realm of familiar, trusting ties was a place of danger where women needed to exercise continuous caution:

Be careful; the times are cruel. I very much want you to think about how in our extremely difficult times, a time of cruelty, crime—this doesn't mean for you to be afraid. No, you should walk with your head lifted high. You should foresee situations, and those you might find yourself in at the last minute. In the evening when you return home from visiting friends, from the disco late, always think that you could await a rape. The times are such that you hear all around not erotica but pornography: in films, in books, in low-level magazines. Therefore everything is filled with sexual tension. And sexual violence is not the desire, so to speak, for sexual satisfaction. And don't think that it's someone who really wants "to screw," [that he] jumps out of a car and pulls someone in from out of a group of defenseless girls. It's not that. It's violence on the *lichnost'*, it reflects a deep injury [*ushcherbnosti*] from early childhood, a difficult, difficult thing. It's a psychopathology, a cruelty, a feeling of power that he can't realize in other spheres of his life. . . . Always be careful. Better to protect yourself than to find yourself in danger, but that's for another lecture, we're out of time now.

Igor Mikhailovich advocated modes of caring for the self that would ensure good health without requiring absolute sexual restraint. He urged young women to be connected to others and responsible to them, but also to remain cautious about the possibility of being victimized by manipulative and violent men. This contrasted sharply with the messages of Anastasia Pavlovna and other gynecologists, who portrayed women with numerous partners as promiscuous, and blamed those who contracted disease as utterly degraded. In their views, warding off the dangers of society required personal moral fortitude, but these providers offered few behavioral skills or communicative strategies for negotiating with others and protecting oneself in situations of danger. Virtuous, upright, and cultured women, they implied, never got into positions where strategies of negotiation would be necessary.

I opened this chapter with a quandary: why did health educators aim to cultivate individual kinds of moral change, rather than raising people's political consciousness and urging social activism to realize their health needs? I suggest several reasons for their rejection of politics as a means of change. First, a didactic approach to patient education was a familiar practice, an element of the Soviet policy that both weakened expert power through deprofessionalization and emphasized it by symbolically valuing expertise. Second, the focus on moral education responded in locally legitimate ways to nationalist campaigns attacking sex education and family planning as furthering Russia's population decline. As nationalists pursued political forms of struggle—submitting petitions to end government funding of family planning, drafting legislation to criminalize abortion, and campaigning against sex education (Ballaeva 1998; Bateneva 1997; Semenov 1996)—they placed health educators on the defensive. To seem legitimate, discourses on sexuality needed to address culturally prevalent anxieties about population. They had to reassert moral boundaries and claim to strengthen family life and reproductive potential. Calls for changes in individual behavior, it seemed, could best realize these goals.

At the same time, in examining sex education lectures ethnographically, I found a diversity of approaches and a range of moral imperatives for individualizing change. While gynecologist-educators urged increasing the discipline of patient obedience, psychologists encouraged patient self-knowledge, strategies of protection, and a view of sexual pleasure as normal and necessary. The latter group imagined themselves as cultivating an individualized, rather than collectivist, subjectivity, and stressed the importance of caring for the self as a matter of personal needs, not as a sacrificial duty to the larger society.

Yet for those providers aiming to develop *lichnost'* as a means of transcending the effects of Soviet state power, it seemed even more paradoxical that my questions about political activism were met with disinterest or objections. I felt strongly that "truly" overcoming Soviet forms of disempowerment would require citizen political empowerment, engaging with the state to demand changes.

Psychologist-educators responded to my suggestions by arguing that the political sphere, like society generally, continued to be seen as a site of corruption, disease, and moral pollution. Like many other Russians, they claimed that despite the breakdown of the Soviet state, little had changed in terms of the actual workings of state/bureaucratic politics. Democracy had not led them to feel empowered to make demands on their legislators or influence policymakers; together with market reforms, it had increased their economic and legal vulnerability. Professionally, they felt neglected by the disinvestments in public health and completely distrusted local and national officials. Speaking in 1995, Paulina Aleksandrovna raised the specter of the destruction and violence undertaken in Chechnya to argue that the post-Soviet government was simply reproducing practices typical of its totalitarian predecessors: following anti-humanistic, undemocratic policies with little regard for the needs and priorities of ordinary citizens. In neither of her social positions—as a professional or a citizen—did she feel she had real access to political influence or an opportunity to reshape political agendas without becoming mired in corruption herself. Her sense of agency, as a consequence, remained located in individual behavior and interpersonal relations. If provider-educators' formulas eschewed collective mobilization and American style "consciousness-raising," but pursued social change by reviving professional authority, that was not all they did. Within a broader social context perceived as physically dangerous and morally uncertain, such educators also struggled to envision and expand certain forms of personal empowerment. I have demonstrated how some, such as Igor Mikhailovich and Paulina Aleksandrovna, forged a model of the professional expert as resource, rather than didactic authoritarian. In this way, they conveyed their vision that the ills Russians faced were not, ultimately, due to their individual failings, but were the results of a state or governmental system that failed to provide opportunities and resources for people to realize their material, informational, and cultural needs. Some educators who held with this view did not limit their educational activities to patients, but conducted moral re-education to cultivate the importance of *lichnost'* among providers as well. Igor Mikhailovich ran monthly group sessions with the obstetrician-gynecologists at his clinic to help them reflect on and refine their approaches with patients. In using his psychotherapy skills with his colleagues, he encouraged them to understand both their patients and themselves as *lichnosti*. To promote a renewed form of professional power, Igor Mikhailovich told his colleagues:

> In principle, you work for a client, you serve a person for his health [*ty sluzhish' cheloveku dlia ego zdorov'ia*], so why should your personal opinions lead you to think [about a patient], "Oh, you're a fool, you're a nobody [*nichtozhestvo*], you, ugh, you're having sex with whoever fell your way, you're carrying contagion. . . ." You understand? A girl can't be reproached for being a certain way [*nel'zia ee uprekat' v tom shto ona v dannyi moment takaia*], for who she sleeps with, or what she does. That's her deep problem.
>
> A gynecologist can have a totally different mentality than a client. But as I see it, the doctor, first and foremost, must not say the word "must" [*dolzhen*]. Because a person must decide what to do himself [*dolzhen-to sam chelovek samomu sebe*]. Your task is to assist the person to consciously understand that it's their situation and their health, it's not up to [the doctor]. A person takes responsibility for himself [not like in] the Soviet, old system [where people said,] "He owes me," [or] "I must [do something]. . . ." If a person doesn't take responsibility for himself, but waits for something from me, like manna from heaven, you can consider him a goner. He must fight for his life, he must make himself healthy for his own salvation [*dlia samospaseniia*].

Lubov' Anatolevna, a gynecologist in her mid thirties, also worked on developing her colleagues' appreciation of patients' *lichnosti,* by training them to conduct contraceptive counseling as a means of reducing abortions. She agreed that encouraging contraceptive use required expert involvement in women's lives. At the same time, however, her efforts to train physicians to offer contraceptive services involved more than just providing physicians with scientifically accurate information. She sought to change physicians' attitudes toward their patients, to help them create trusting relationships with women—in her words, to *morally educate doctors:*

> Sometimes I see a woman leave the family planning office with contraceptives, but I see in her face that she doesn't believe the doctor. I'll ask her, "Are you going to use these contraceptives? Tell me honestly, because if not, then maybe we can find some-

thing else for you that you will use." Then we may even go back and talk to the doctor. The doctor may have no idea whatsoever that the woman didn't understand or trust her. I tell the doctors, "You have to listen to the woman, give her a chance to talk, to find out her problems and concerns, or else she'll leave here and won't use what you give her." The doctors don't understand this for the most part. Our system didn't teach doctors to do this. They just get a patient and say, "Take this pill, drink this, do that," but they don't give them a chance to ask any questions and don't have any interactions with the woman. The women then walk away and don't follow the doctor's directions. . . . I try very hard to explain to the doctors how to deal with women, but it's difficult. I have to morally educate [*vospitivat'*] the doctors, that's the most important thing, so that they'll be able to reach the women.

Like Paulina Aleksandrovna and Igor Mikhailovich, Lubov' Anatolevna interpreted the problems surrounding women's reproductive health as symptoms of the social diseases wrought on the nation by the Soviet system. She saw abortion use as a sign that all kinds of interpersonal relations—including between doctors and patients—had become distorted under the Soviet era. Pervasive illness and compromised health were not merely physical, she argued; the nation was suffering from a diseased social order stemming from the disrespect of individuality [*lichnost'*]:

Our Soviet system didn't focus on the question of personality/individuality [*lichnost'*]. This was a major part of the problem. Women didn't see their children as needing to be developed, as in need of attention to help them develop and learn. We became a closed, introverted [*zamknutye*] people. We don't open ourselves up. We don't relate to each other.

By working to promote contraceptive use over abortion, and by training providers to consider women's individual needs and desires, Lubov' Anatolevna was pursuing social change both in personhood and in the accepted model of professional power. That Igor Mikhailovich and Lubov' Anatolevna promoted the notion of *lichnost'* among professionals as well as patients leads me to see their work as different from the efforts of their colleagues in several ways. They saw poor intercommunication, domestic gender conflicts, ignorance about the body and sexuality, the habitual use of abortion, and the underdevelopment of *lichnost'* as destructive effects of the Soviet system on people's attitudes, behaviors, and interpersonal relations—not simply as individual failings and moral deficits. They considered moral education a valuable, pragmatic way of overcoming lingering effects of the state and socialist past. Consequently, these educators aimed to increase individual empowerment, if in selective ways. Changing persons and selves enabled these providers to target the traces of the bureaucracy and Soviet ideology that they saw invading Russians' personal lives, and struggle against them.

Psychologist-educators' faith that a renewed sense of *lichnost'* enables autonomy from the state, and their attempts to privatize human experiences in intimate zones and practices, recalls the relationship between the private sphere and individual "freedom" central to American liberalism. There are, however, some unexpected twists in Russian educational practices that underscore the local character of the emerging public-private split and raise questions about the limits of such idealized personal autonomy. Psychologists' advocacy of masturbation offers a key example. On the one hand, they aimed to demystify and normalize masturbation as a private experience in order to empower young people and enhance their sense of freedom from collectivist discourses and obligations. Simultaneously, however, the lectures achieved this "empowerment" through a very *public* form of openness and, in Igor Mikhailovich's terms, a rather prescriptive language: "I recommend this very intimate thing—although each to her own—in principle, a woman must caress herself." Advocating for sexual practices in this way retains a sense that one's bodily habits are the concern of the public, or at least of interested professionals. The impossibility of a completely "private" sphere emerges again in Igor Mikhailovich's discussions, when he advises young women to carry condoms with them as a means of ensuring safe sex, but immediately acknowledges that mothers routinely go through daughters' purses. Monitoring continues, in both professional and domestic spheres, but the privatizing ideal of an independent Self retains a powerful resonance.

The selfhood known as *lichnost'* that Russian providers promoted, finally, was quite distinct from the self-sufficient individual of the American imagination. Rather than conceived of as an autonomous "individual," *lichnost'* is best rendered through the concept of a fully mature self-in-relation, a person with self-knowledge, self-respect, and the ability to engage in ethical relations with others—relations that similarly respect other selves' unique needs, and *seek their fulfillment.* Women in particular were instructed to develop *lichnosti* capable of caring for others: educators' imperatives for women's hygiene and sexual and reproductive behavior ultimately served the good of their male partners or unborn babies. By linking *lichnost'* to the profoundly salient notion of compulsory reciprocity, educators found the concept flexible enough to promote a host of agendas. They also rendered tame its dangerous potential to signify unlimited freedom.[12]

PART 2
Practices

FOUR

Taking Responsibility for Ourselves

ALLA'S ENCOUNTER

It was a typical afternoon in May, the time when physicians on the pre-natal ward took the medical histories of women who had been admit-ted that day, and examined them. I sat down as doctors Natalia Borisovna and Nina Petrovna were commiserating on the large number of women who had arrived. Nina Petrovna suggested that they had probably been waiting to admit themselves until after the recent holidays.

Natalia Borisovna motioned to the woman standing outside her office door to enter, and using the familiar form of address [*ty*], said to her gen-tly, "Come, my dear [*moia khoroshaia*], I'll examine you."

Entering the room with barren, pale walls and uncomfortable, decrepit furniture, Alla sat down in the rickety, vacant chair. She appeared at an early stage of pregnancy, probably only in the second trimester. Natalia Borisovna opened her chart and saw that the prenatal clinic had referred her here after failing to hear a fetal heartbeat. This was interpreted as a sign of potentially serious trouble because Alla had previously suffered two mis-carriages during or close to the second trimester. The situation was thus urgent: they needed to diagnose the problem quickly and hopefully could save the pregnancy. To begin this process, the physicians attempted to gain as many additional details of her medical history as possible and sought to have Alla elaborate on her previous miscarriages.

Without giving any other greetings or introducing herself, Natalia Borisovna began immediately taking Alla's history: "Early childhood sick-ness? They've written here nephritis; have you had anything else?"

"I had nephritis again in '92 and hepatitis in '94."

Natalia Borisovna plunged into the interview, jumping rapidly from questions arising from the woman's medical file to a series of standard questions asked of every woman in the intake interview: "Were you in the hospital? . . . Have you had any contact with TB? . . . It says here you had jaundice. How old is your husband? . . . Is he healthy? . . . At what age did your menstrual period begin? . . . How many days long is your cycle? . . . Is it regular? . . . When did you first become sexually active? . . . Have you had any gynecological sicknesses? . . . This is your first pregnancy?"

"I had a miscarriage."

"What happened?"

"It just happened [*prosto tak*]."

Upon hearing this answer, Natalia Borisovna grew frustrated, and her tone became aggressive: "How can it 'just happen'?"

With her voice so timid it was barely above a whisper, Alla admitted, "I don't know, the water broke."

"Did they do curettage?"

"Yes."

"When were you discharged? [pause] How many days were you in the hospital?"

"I don't remember."

Natalia Borisovna, overtly exasperated, sped up the tempo of her questions. The result was that the "interview" became a mixture of scolding and interrogation, in which she often did not wait for the woman to answer.

"How can you not remember? You're a young girl, you were there seven days, did you have an inflamed uterus?"

"I don't know."

"Did they give you antibiotics?"

"Yes."

"What'd they say to you? Maybe there was a fever?"

Observing the exchange, Nina Petrovna offered Natalia Borisovna an idea about what happened. She made no eye contact with the woman patient. "It was most likely a miscarriage that took place out of the hospital."

Natalia Borisovna continued the interrogation. "When was your second pregnancy?" Then, without waiting for an answer, she repeated an earlier question: "When you had the miscarriage, did they do curettage?"

"Yes."

At this point, Natalia Borisovna addressed the woman by name for the first time in the interview, using the affectionate diminutive form: "Allochka, when were you discharged? And this is now your third pregnancy?"

"Yes."

"Do you need this pregnancy? When you came to the prenatal clinic, why didn't you ask, why didn't you get interested? You had a miscarriage at twenty-two weeks; this shouldn't happen in a woman who is young and healthy. Did you ask the doctor, go to him and ask, 'Why did I have a miscarriage?' Usually after someone has a miscarriage, they tell you, or they do a psychological examination. Why didn't you say to them, 'Please tell me why this happened'?"

Alla's face betrayed no hint of her emotions, but her laconic responses seemed to me obvious signs of fear and intimidation. "They told me I had a miscarriage, and that was all."

Natalia Borisovna persisted, first trying a gentle tone, and then letting her frustration get the better of her: "There had to be a reason. Did you have any blood transfusions?"

Alla shook her head to indicate she had not.

Looking at the chart, the doctor noted, "You're at twenty-six weeks— if you have a miscarriage now, will you be interested?"

Speaking quietly, Alla stated simply, "I am."

Natalia Borisovna persisted with her questions. "Do you have any allergies? . . . Have you been sick in the last two weeks? . . . Is anyone at home sick? . . . Have you gone out of town recently? . . . I see you began prenatal care at eight weeks. How much weight should a pregnant woman gain?"

"About eight kilos," Alla answered, providing the correct response.

Yet Natalia Borisovna gave her no credit for this, but warned her of her impending danger. "You've already gained this. In the second part of the pregnancy a woman gains most of her weight. Now what do we do with you?"

Natalia Borisovna continued by interrogating Alla on her eating and (nonalcoholic) drinking habits, to ascertain whether she was consuming amounts of liquid the doctor considered excessive.[1] After calculating Alla's daily intake to be about one and a half liters of liquid, she announced that the patient, who suffered from "chronic nephritis," needed to be restricted to one liter per day, including liquids from fruits and vegetables, in order to lose some weight.

For the first time in the entire exchange, Alla initiated a statement. "Last week there was a lot of movement, now it's stopped and I got scared."

"Do you have any discomfort?"

"None. [pause] But the doctor couldn't find the heartbeat."

"At twenty-some weeks, you usually can't hear anything, you can't hear the fetus's heart."

"My doctor heard it before."

Nina Petrovna joined in again. "What's your doctor's name?"

"Tatiana? Tatiana Aleksandrovna maybe?"

Natalia Borisovna frowned and explained, "At twenty-two weeks you can't hear; it's absurd, it was only your pulse. They can only tell with the ultrasound."[2]

"I myself can feel the movements."

"Have you read any books about pregnancy?"

"No."

Natalia Borisovna responded sarcastically, "Good going."

It was Nina Petrovna who took over then, interceding with an angry tirade. "There's stuff all over the place, as much as you want, just go and find it. You don't even need to have a desire. You got pregnant, what are you thinking? How are you preparing for the birth? You need to know how the pregnancy progresses, where the organs are. It's your pregnancy, and this should interest every woman, both out of simple curiosity and more."

Natalia Borisovna picked up on her colleague's sense of disgust, responding to Nina Petrovna as if Alla was not in the room. "She's had two miscarriages, the first at twenty-two weeks and the second at ten weeks. She doesn't know or need to know [anything]. It's the third pregnancy and she hasn't read any books, she doesn't need anything. Oh, I can't take it anymore, I can't take it [*Ia bol'she ne mogu*]."

Nina Petrovna then took charge of the interview. With the medical history concluded, she escorted Alla to the examining room across the hall. A few minutes later, Nina Petrovna yelled from the examining room, "She's at twenty-one weeks now, as she estimates. Her aorta is so strong, that's what we feel, her aorta!"

Speaking then to Alla, she instructed, "Don't drink anything more. Go relax, lie down in your room. Your aorta is so strong, the beat goes through your whole body."

Alla was allowed to leave then, and promptly escaped to her room. As with many patients whom the doctors encounter, Alla seemed to know very little about the details of her medical history. Yet instead of recognizing the failure of the health care system to ensure adequate records of the patients' history and to provide clear-cut information to each woman about her condition and the procedures undertaken on her, they blamed the patient herself. Highlighting Alla's perceived indifference as the core of these problems, Natalia Borisovna sank into despair over her own plight as a physician. "I can't take it anymore," she exclaimed, stating she had reached the limit of her patience for working with women having "such a low level."

In reaching a diagnosis (and finally asking the patient herself how far along she was), Nina Petrovna found that Alla was at an earlier stage of pregnancy than her chart had listed. Consequently, the inaudible fetal heartbeat was not a cause for concern, because "at the earliest," she explained, "the fetal heart is not audible until twenty-four weeks. Moreover, if the woman's skinny, if the placenta's not right in front, and even later on, if the heartbeat is weak, sometimes you'll only hear the woman's aorta, and then every so often, you can hear a weak, faint beat of the baby, but even then not always."

This exchange was typical of intake interviews. Since physicians sat together interviewing patients in a single room, the number of doctors a woman might engage with varied, a situation that fragmented care yet further. In their encounters with physicians, patients usually restricted their comments to laconic, polite responses. I rarely heard informal conversations between physicians and patients; the few times I witnessed women attempting to chat casually, their efforts were rebuffed. It was only with women who immediately identified themselves as health care providers, and whose charts confirmed their professional status, that immediate rapport emerged. "Despite being dressed in this nightgown and robe, I'm actually one of you," such women would convey, knowing intuitively the important social bond this would create. "I understand your plight, don't lump me with *those* patients," their eyes asserted.

Alla's encounter with the prenatal ward doctors thus illustrates common dynamics of provider-patient relations at what I call maternity hospital No. 5, and other health care institutions in St. Petersburg during the mid 1990s. Twenty-one years old, recently married, and with a vocational education, Alla was typical of many of this hospital's patients, who generally had few economic or social resources. While Alla's medical records left major gaps in information that Natalia Borisovna and Nina Petrovna needed, they attacked her for not knowing all the details of her past experiences. They saw Alla's demeanor as a typical product of the Soviet system, which, they felt, encouraged indifference about one's health and insubordination toward expert authority. My sense is that Alla feared hospital staff as typical agents of the bureaucratic state system, known for acting out of self-interest and disregarding their obligations to help the women they were employed to serve.

But I do not know exactly what Alla thought. As I observed her intake interview and many others like it on a daily basis during fieldwork, I felt at once compelled to hear women's sides of the story and profoundly reluctant to intervene in their lives with further questioning or prodding. Draped in the white coat of bureaucratic power, I had a degree of authority over women patients, and thus a request to answer my questions automatically carried with it a degree of coercion. I surmised that women might fear speaking openly with me given my ties to the doctors and hospital administrators (visible in the white coat I was required to wear). But they might also fear that refusing to speak with me could jeopardize their health care. I consequently needed to approach women patients with the utmost of care, to convey to them that talking with me was completely voluntary and that no negative consequences would occur if they preferred not to. On more than one occasion, women like Alla whom I approached in the maternity hospital after such conflicted interactions with the doctors averted my eyes altogether, or agreed to an interview with evident reluctance. They usually did not say, "No, I really don't want to talk to you." They registered their refusal instead through symbolic resistance alone—gestures of disinterest, disdain, silence. Feeling immensely invasive, I would smile and retreat, saying, "You know, never mind, it's not necessary," and with an embarrassed look of apology, I would stammer, "Thank you anyway," or "Good luck to you." My uncertainty as to whether I could avoid coercion and create the trust necessary for patients to express themselves frequently led me to avoid following up with women whom I first observed in intake interviews. On the other hand, I knew that my task in Russia was to hear all sides of the story of reproductive health care and to uncover the voices of those most muted in public discussions of the problems and potential solutions to the reproductive health crisis. One solution I took was to seek out women patients whom I had not already encountered when sitting together with health care providers. This enabled me to introduce myself and my project without appearing as closely connected to hospital staff (although sometimes doctors accompanied me to women's rooms with the aim of "encouraging" women to participate). In time, as I increasingly witnessed conflicts and humiliations during intake interviews, I did seek out these women patients, trying with gentleness and understanding to offer them the chance to speak about their experiences in the hospital. I began by explaining that the purpose of my book was to help English-speaking readers understand Russia and to enter into more effective relationships to improve Russians' health care, not to judge whether or not Russians were "doing things right." By acknowledging that I had seen painful, conflict-ridden interactions and wanted to hear women's perspectives on their experiences in the maternity hospital, I tried to convey that my white coat did not determine my stance and that I aimed to obtain a variety of views in an open-minded and sympathetic way. Finally, by promising that I would keep our discussion entirely confidential and would change all names in my future writing, I attempted to alleviate their worries about sharing their ideas, and perhaps to begin a relationship.

Fortunately, many women eagerly agreed to share their stories with me. Admitted to the prenatal ward on bed rest to save an endangered pregnancy or to wait for labor to begin in the last days of their pregnancy, they had time to talk. My accented Russian was intriguing, and the opportunity to talk with an American seemed an interesting distraction from the tiresome hospital routine. Several women invited me to visit them at home after the birth. I met women of different ages, educational levels, marital status, geographical background, and ethnicity, interviewed many of them several times, and maintained long-term contact with several women over the course of this research.

A key insight of my research is that clashes between providers and patients in the mid 1990s were a key component of the way each side struggled to ensure healthy childbearing. Despite the feminized character of this institution—only two or three male doctors worked there during the entire seven years of my study—there was no inkling of gender-based solidarity between providers and patients. Provider worlds and patient domains constituted interconnected but distinct microcosms, with each group striving desperately—often against the other—to realize positive, healthy outcomes for mother and child.

In laypersons' imagination and experience, the health care institution was a site where the rules and practices governing social exchange were frighteningly ambiguous, and those in power seemed as likely to flout accepted norms of interpersonal decency as they were to uphold them. Women resented the rude, aggressive behavior they encountered from health care providers. Yet such actions were not unfamiliar. Women described them to me as typical of "our system," a concept that referred to the controlling, coercive dimensions of state power that became perceptible in everyday bureaucratic interactions.

Many of the stories I tell in this part of the book are therefore painful. In settings expected to be sites of healing and caring, the pervasive vulnerability affecting both providers and patients often gave rise to hostility and cruelty. I present these accounts not in order to perpetuate false stereotypes of Russians as steeped in authoritarian behaviors or as incorrigibly corrupt. My goal in fact is just the opposite: to show how the socialist health care system, with its hypocritical treatment of physician power, combined with the new inequities and injustices of market reforms, entangled providers and patients in systemic conflict. Moreover, I strive to demonstrate how women on both sides of the struggle strategized against these forces, to the extent they were able. Their conflicts turned medical power into a site of intense negotiation over the shared desire to create a benevolent, authoritative form of expertise.

If some women approached me with caution, there was also the possibility of alienating hospital staff with this research. Sometime after beginning fieldwork, I learned how the hospital's chief doctor, Nelly Ivanovna, informed her staff about my project. She warned them that they had better be on their best behavior since "an inspector" would be coming to

observe them. By the time I found out about the remark, I already understood that this threat was typical of the chief doctor's disciplinary tactics.
Fortunately, when I first met Natalia Borisovna and other staff, I immediately explained that my goal was not to judge their compliance with WHO
recommendations, but to understand their and their patients' experiences
of post-Soviet reforms. I would convey their ideas back to WHO and
other interested foreigners, in order to improve our efforts to help. The
providers were intrigued by the idea of having a Russian-speaking American to talk with—and, no doubt, about. They also seemed to appreciate
my anthropological positioning as a novice regarding their lives. The physicians explained their schedule to me and told me I could come "to work"
any morning after the staff meeting and rounds. I was welcome to sit with
them as they filled out their paperwork, had tea and lunch, and conducted
their afternoon admitting consultations with new patients. On Tuesdays
before lunch, Natalia Borisovna, chief of the prenatal ward, or Nina Petrovna, chief of the gynecological unit for women with complications in
early terms of pregnancy, gave lectures to women about childbirth and
breastfeeding. Tuesday and Thursday afternoons, visiting hours officially
took place. Also on these days, women from the community could consult
with hospital physicians about giving birth there in the future. I was welcome to attend any of these, too.

Natalia Borisovna and Nina Petrovna quickly initiated me into the
casual and open atmosphere they had between themselves and most other
health providers in the hospital. Lunch was a crucial reprieve from the
burdens of the day's work, and they used the time to socialize, blow off
steam, and gain each other's advice about various problems. Tightly packed
in the cramped gynecological unit office, they covered its small plastic
table with a flowered vinyl cloth and servings of the two-course institutional meal of soup followed by meat and potatoes fed to all the hospital.
To make the atmosphere more cozy, and the meal more satisfying, the
doctors brought extras from home. Cucumbers (fresh or pickled), a beet
and potato salad, a kiwi or some apples, and perhaps a hunk of cheese or
salami, were added to the table, making a daily potluck gathering. With
the door closed tightly, the doctors re-enacted arguments with patients
and administrators and discussed their anxieties about ongoing patient
cases. Sometimes the issues were heated, as when a twenty-five-year-old
woman giving birth to her third child by planned caesarean requested that
the doctors also tie her tubes. "There's no way I will do this!" Natalia
Borisovna bellowed for the entire lunch, enraged at what she perceived
was the woman's lack of foresight about her possible future, and fearful of
the potential punishments she herself might endure for performing this
operation, should the woman later change her mind.[3] On calmer days, the

providers spoke of their family problems and consulted each other about where to buy certain products cheaply. Often they helped each other fill in crossword puzzles, planned birthday celebrations for other hospital personnel, and with laughter and ridicule read each other magazine surveys about men and sex. After drinking tea and washing the dishes in the cold water of the office sink, Natalia Borisovna would heat up her curling iron to fix her hair, and Nina Petrovna would join her at the small mirror to touch up her lipstick. Throughout the time I was present, the physicians made concerted efforts to make me feel included in their company. Whenever I failed to understand a medical term or a joke, I was encouraged to ask for clarification. The acceptance the doctors showed me soon extended into after-clinic hours, too. Both Natalia Borisovna and Nina Petrovna invited me to their homes for dinner and took me on several sightseeing trips around the city. Their concern for the success of my project, and their friendship, touched me greatly. They left me with a profound sense of obligation to represent them fairly.

A central requirement of my fieldwork thus became developing trusting relationships with both providers and patients, in order to understand their intertwined plights and their conflicts. One more person whose help was invaluable for this was Karina, a member of the hospital's housecleaning staff who became a very dear friend. Neither expert nor patient, she was a liminal figure in this institution. She was also an extraordinarily sensitive, intelligent, and caring person able to see every incident from multiple perspectives. My own observations, conversations, and interviews with providers and patients, and my discussions with Karina during or after fieldwork, form the basis for my description, first of patients' strategies for ensuring healthy pregnancies and births, and then of providers' efforts.

As Karina and I talked, I came to see that both sides, ironically, described the core of their conflicts by asserting that the other failed to take responsibility for reproductive health. For patients, this failure emerged when clinicians at the prenatal center refused to treat women themselves but passed them off to maternity hospital doctors, essentially requiring extended and seemingly unnecessary hospital stays. It emerged again in their encounters with maternity hospital staff, who seemed to disregard the specifics of each woman's case and instead prescribed all possible medicines and took all possible precautions to protect *themselves*—at what felt like the expense of women's health. The worst expressions of this irresponsibility involved aggressive behavior intended to intimidate and dominate patients. Women described these behaviors as signs that "our system"— with its hostility and unreliability—inhabited those persons supposed to be the caregivers. To combat this dangerous force, many women withheld trust from anyone associated with the health care institution, and spoke instead of trying to take responsibility for themselves. They did not, notably, imagine this move to be aimed at enhancing their "equality." Most frequently, women framed their desire for change by asserting the need for a "higher level of professionalism" among experts.

Doctors had very different views of the problem. They considered women en masse to be apathetic about their health, indifferent to expert advice and knowledge, and fatally irresponsible toward their future children. They felt justified in this impression when they repeatedly caught pregnant women smoking in the bathroom, or climbing on unstable chairs to reach out the windows to talk to their husbands, risking catching a cold at best or falling to their deaths at worst. Doctors blamed the entire Soviet system for teaching citizens to disregard their health while expecting doctors to cure them miraculously; and they blamed that same governmental system for creating structural conditions in health care that denied experts the full range of support they needed. Poor material conditions and waning resources frustrated doctors daily, as they confronted dwindling supplies of antibiotics and a lack of hot water. Providers were called to participate in tasks well beyond their professional profiles, for there was no money in the hospital budget for trimming the bushes or bailing water after a severe flood. Doctors' salaries barely covered a month's food needs for a family, and staying in medicine increasingly seemed a luxury available only to those with other sources of financial support. But the problems were not only economic and technical. In the words of one very kind, very tired male physician, the Soviet public health system had structured "collective irresponsibility" [*kollektivnaia bezotvetstvennost'*] at its core, by fragmenting care, preventing specialists with different profiles from readily consulting each other, and leaving each caregiver to participate in only one tiny aspect of the overall process of a woman's pregnancy and birth.

Providers never admitted that they, personally, had become part of "our system," a statement tantamount to admitting one's professional integrity was compromised. They saw the negative personal characteristics enabled by "our system"—indifference and selfishness—in others, from their patients to their superiors and some colleagues. Each individual experienced herself as suffering at the hands of "our system," not empowered by it. And if many providers responded to this failing structure by striving to compensate for it with individualizing forms of action based on their personal dedication and perseverance, this did not necessarily lead them to recognize women's victimization. Providers often worked to enforce patients' sense of "responsibility" through desperate, futile practices —demanding respect for expert authority and coercing compliance. I believe that these patterned forms of hostility in clinic interactions derived from the contradictory combination of Russia's profound veneration of expertise, on the one hand, and the socialist policy of deprofessionalization, which eliminated medical workers' economic and political power, on the other. Doctors were left groping for a means of experiencing the social status they felt certain they deserved.

But this structural, political-economic explanation of provider-patient conflicts was not part of Russians' everyday understandings and practices. If laypersons and experts considered the lack of responsibility structured into the state system as the foremost obstacle to health, both groups coped with this failure by trying to assume responsibility themselves, and demanding that others do the same. These attempts occurred as providers and patients considered themselves as individual agents able to act apart from "the system," and also as they bonded in informal ways with acquaintances and close friends to personalize the anonymous, bureaucratic health care encounter. In either case, the consistent effort to bypass the official health care system precluded both an organized political alliance based on a common gender identity between doctors and patients and an effort by either group to struggle as a collectivity to defend their interests. When I shared my analysis that physicians' lack of political-economic power over their work lives and health policymaking created a painful contradiction for them by betraying their sense of entitlement to social authority, Natalia Borisovna listened attentively. Yet when I told how physicians in the U.S. gain substantial power through organizing themselves in professional associations that lobby (and financially support) political representatives, she responded dismissively, as if I had just described an exotic phenomenon unreal for Russian doctors. Another gynecologist, Liuba, insisted that "this would NEVER be possible in Russia!" "They'll never give us power!" she boomed, unable to imagine her profession independently organizing to demand power itself.

The structural obstacles known as "our system" seemed utterly entrenched in society, and ultimately unassailable. The pragmatic kind of strategy laypersons and experts devised for coping with their daily constraints thus suggests a continuity between socialist and "post-socialist" life: despite the advent of "democratic" political processes, collective dilemmas—*even when recognized as such*—seemed resolvable only through piecemeal, individualized, and/or personalized tactics for moral change.

PATIENTS' STRATEGIES

When arriving at the hospital to "lie" on the prenatal ward for observation or actually give birth, a woman entered the institution through a side entrance known as the *priemnyi pokoi,* the admitting room. In this small cubicle, a pregnant woman began her bout of negotiations with the state health care institution as she handed over her prenatal file, was instructed to undress and shower, and got stripped of any nail polish, jewelry, and pubic hair. She was then given an enema, was dressed in a hospital gown and robe, and, having been officially "prepared," was brought to the prenatal ward or the delivery room. She entered the admitting room alone. Her relatives would later approach the hospital staff through a neighboring door, which housed the information desk and the site for dropping off packages of food for patients upstairs. In the many months of the year that the chief doctor suspended visiting hours ("Without the funds to hire a security guard, we can't protect the women against drunken husbands," Karina explained), the information desk became a family's sole liaison to the seemingly impenetrable world their relative had entered.

Once settled into the prenatal ward, women became acquainted with the institution's daily routine: breakfast in the communal dining room, doctors' rounds, educational lectures or films, lunch, an afternoon rest period, and, when not cancelled, visiting hours twice weekly in the afternoon, followed by dinner. Toilets and showers were on the hallway, equipped with nothing but the machinery. Toilet paper and soap were strictly bring-your-own. There was a television in the hallway lounge where some women gathered to watch popular soap operas such as the American production *Santa Barbara,* but many women remained in their rooms most of the day. Some spoke with their husbands on the pay phone in the corridor; others hollered out the windows of their rooms to communicate with relatives, who were standing on the ground three flights below, often in the cold.

Many women patients whom I spoke with expressed confidence in their ability to care for themselves and suspicion of the motives and competence of maternity home staff. Women on the prenatal ward for "observation" and "rest" in the early stages of pregnancy often complained that the doctors "aren't doing anything for me," "aren't treating me." They felt frustrated that doctors failed to convey the precise nature of their conditions and only vaguely described the treatments they were prescribing. Women told of reading old gynecological textbooks they had found in friends' homes to gain information; many went to lectures at prenatal clinics too. They resented being kept in the hospital for days on end merely in order to be given pills. Olga, a single, thirty-six-year-old engineer in her second trimester, insisted, "I could take this medicine myself, at home. Nina Petrovna told me [imitating a threatening voice], 'You're not able to take care of yourself!' They want to insure themselves thoroughly, and [therefore] overprotect themselves. But I want to be discharged, to be out in the fresh air. I know my body, and I know that staying here in this small room, with no air, it's bad." The doctors' reproaches to Olga for giving birth in her mid thirties further convinced her that their own fears and desire "to avoid responsibility" for her case led them to prescribe unnecessary treatments and medical surveillance.

As women spoke about problems of the public health system, they drew connections to the overall system of power based in state socialism that persisted in post-Soviet conditions, especially for the many people unable to pay for the emerging fee-for-service care. Notably, patients did not blame these problems on particular staff members. While Olga had a negative encounter with Nina Petrovna, for example, she told me, "You can't blame a specific doctor, it's our system. The old system that was in place for 70 years . . ." "Our system," as Olga described it, was the complex bureaucracy of state socialism. Without money to buy potentially better choices, she felt her tactics for overcoming this system were limited. Feeling alone, vulnerable, and angry, Olga had the solace of her sense of personal moral integrity—her readiness to accept responsibility for herself.

Highly educated and traveled Russians told me that they never went to the doctor for routine preventive care, and upon getting pregnant (and deciding to keep the pregnancy), waited as long as possible to begin prenatal care. [4] "Why should I go—so they can send me running all over the city to do tests?" came the blunt retort from Margarita, an English language teacher and translator. This was not only a matter of inconvenience; she insisted that the doctors were poorly trained, unmotivated, rude, and indifferent. Without understanding the precise structural arrangements shaping the hospital's "collective irresponsibility," including the fragmented division of labor separating women's care into different segments of birth, Margarita's and other women's lifetime experiences led them to expect that some kind of systemic barriers stood in the way of quality care. The fact that the precise structural problems were not understood added, of course, to women's sense of vulnerability and their inability to strategize effectively to overcome these problems.

Many grounded their skepticism on providers' eternally low salaries: patients feared that with no economic incentive for providing good care, providers had no moral incentive to do so, either. Others saw in providers a more complex set of constraints that had resulted in a feeling of professional exhaustion, an inability to struggle against mounting obstacles that gradually became expressed as indifference. Karina told me that when a provider had lost her ability to be gentle and caring, when her face had hardened, it was a sign that she had been beaten down by life [*zabitaia zhizn'iu*]. Providers like this had succumbed to a lifetime of burdens and stress, to repeated painful workplace frustrations compounded with personal tragedies. "Our system," Karina and several patients explained, had created the conditions where such experiences were terribly common. It created a work environment where authoritarian management styles and poor material conditions placed providers in ethically awkward, compromising positions, such as requiring women to bring their own medications, bed sheets, and disposable gloves for the providers because of the state's failures to adequately fund even "free" maternity care. Following a day of these unpleasant responsibilities, women providers then returned home to face domestic burdens under cramped living conditions with few household amenities, and a second shift of hard labor in housework. If many patients recognized these structural (gendered) dimensions of providers' constraints, they had no way to use this knowledge for improving their situations. It was merely a souring consolation—a sense that the grass was truly *not* greener on the other side.

One patient who agreed to speak with me after I witnessed a conflict she had with the prenatal ward doctors offered similar insights. Elena was thirty-one years old, originally from a provincial city called Nevel' in the district of Pskov, a small city three hours by car from St. Petersburg. For the past eight years, she had been working in the quality control department in a factory that made wood products. She was married and lived in a dorm room. She came to Leningrad in 1986 despite having "a good job" in the library in Nevel', because "a single girl who isn't getting married doesn't have much to do there. So I came to Leningrad, to the woodworking college [*uchilishche*]." She met her husband at the factory, where he was also employed. Although he was from Leningrad, he had been living with his mother, and, she explained to me, there wasn't anywhere for them to live together. "I got a dorm room from the factory, so we have a decent room. Compared with how others live, it's not bad."

I didn't know anything about Elena, however, when she first appeared outside the door of the prenatal ward office, during the afternoon period when doctors wrote up notes from their morning rounds. Nina Petrovna was filling in her patients' files, and I was writing field notes. Elena and two other patients approached the door but stood in the hallway just outside the threshold. She quietly asked Nina Petrovna something about shots; I was sitting rather far from the door and didn't hear the question well. All of a sudden Nina Petrovna turned her body toward the women and enraged, began yelling:

> Your hemoglobin is 96, if you don't want to, don't take it, nobody's forcing you! Do whatever you want, you don't need a medical degree to conceive and raise children. If you don't want to take the shots, fine with me! Don't take them. It's your problem!! But I'm telling you, your cervix is bad, and we must prepare it. If you want to get a blood transfusion with someone else's blood, that's just fine. You'll get donor

blood after having all these complications from giving birth with this low level of hemoglobin. But everyone gets to decide for themselves, it's up to you [*eto delo khoziaiskoe*]!

As Nina Petrovna lurched forward and yelled, her contorted facial expression and threatening tone of voice left little doubt about the message she intended to convey. Her hostile stance asserted, "You're a stupid fool! You should just do what I tell you—but you have the right to be foolish and do what you want. So go ahead, I dare you, take the stupid risk!"

Intimidated by this angry response, Elena and the others backed away even farther from the office door, retreating until they were standing in the middle of the corridor. But they did not give up. Elena looked away from Nina Petrovna to the window at the end of the hallway and meekly muttered, "I want to know what the medicine is and what it is for." Nina Petrovna responded by yelling, "I told you what it is, Spasmolitik." Elena and the two others walked away.

I sat there stunned at Nina Petrovna's ability to go into a rage so easily, and then just as quickly come out of it. After a few minutes had gone by, I asked Nina Petrovna what that had been all about. Now less incensed but still evidently frustrated as she recalled the incident, Nina Petrovna explained: "They don't want to take this medicine. [In a mocking tone] *They want to take responsibility for themselves.*"

"What are you prescribing for them?" I asked.

Without going into detail about each woman's case, she enumerated a range of vitamins they needed to take. "There are several shots, of iron, vitamins B1, B6, B12, and iron with folic acid."

"So they wanted to know about these?" I asked, to clarify what was at stake in this exchange.

Nina Petrovna, exasperated with the encounter (and probably my questions too), again gave a rather vague explanation. More importantly, she refused to concede that the women's inquiries were valid attempts to understand their health needs. Rather, she perceived the questions as attacks on her authority as an expert: "All three of them are prescribed different injections. One doesn't want vitamin B because of the pain of the shot, the other doesn't want vitamin C glucose for placental insufficiency, and the third doesn't want [a pill] to lower the inflammation."

The next day I returned to the maternity hospital and sought out Elena. It was then that I introduced myself and my project to her, explained that I had seen how she had been talked to the day before, and asked to hear her perspective on what happened. I assured her that everything she said to me would be held in confidence, and that her name would be changed in anything I wrote about the encounter.

With a look mixed with caution and intrigue, Elena agreed to speak with me. She began by acknowledging her anger and the sense of injustice she felt at Nina Petrovna's actions the day before: "The way she was yelling at us, 'Fine, don't get treated, do what you want!' Well, you heard it all yourself, I don't have to explain. We came and asked her because there are many rumors that they inject you with all kinds of things. Maybe earlier we didn't want to know things, but now we do."

"Why do you think things have changed? How have they changed?" I asked her.

Elena explained that women no longer revered physicians, but wanted some understanding of their condition and care: "Earlier we thought that doctors were Tsar and God, and we didn't ask anything, there was complete subordination. But now we want to know a bit. Even at the prenatal clinic [the midwife] told us—you should know what's going on. At other maternity homes there are many infections, there is staph, here it's relatively lower."

"I think the doctors feel that the women don't trust them," I offered.

Elena repeated her analysis of the source of provider-patient miscommunication, and then explained that the problem was not universal; there were some providers who managed to be caring and friendly despite the immense difficulties of their work: "No, the doctors expect women to treat them as God and the Tsar. But today, there was a different nurse, she was totally different. She was very nice. She has so many women to take care of, and I'm sure she has a lot of worries and gets overwhelmed, but she was very sweet, nice and understanding. It was totally different."

"The nurse yesterday was different?" I asked.

"Yes," Elena said. "When I asked her what medication she was handing me, she cut me off, saying, 'I don't know anything, the doctor wrote it!' For all these providers, to put it crudely, it's the typical behavior: 'I'm the boss—you're the fool.' I wouldn't say it's everywhere, but it's often. Probably the same with their administration, the head doctor probably yells at them and then it's a whole chain."

I nodded my head vigorously and agreed: "You're absolutely right, they complain about that all the time."

Without a trace of surprise, Elena smiled slightly. "I figured that; it often works that way."

Elena told me about her preparation for birth and the positive experiences she had had prior to this hospital. She found the lectures she had attended at her prenatal clinic very helpful. She remembered specific pieces of advice the midwife gave, from how to deal with the physical process of childbirth to how to cope with the maternity hospital as an institution:

> She told us about birth. She had had a wealth of experiences and had gone abroad, and she told us how they do it all there. She told us what symptoms you have [when

about to give birth], and how to behave, not to be scared. She said it's sort of like a period. She said it's better not to scream, it's bad for the baby. Imagine, if it's hard psychologically when the doctors yell at you, for a baby the yelling is even harder.

The midwife also encouraged Elena to be informed about the medicines and the process, and to feel empowered in childbirth: "She was friendly, and she spoke to us mostly from her own personal experiences. She told us about the names of medicines since doctors want you to know them. And she said to us, 'You have the right to refuse and to sign a document that says you want to leave, even when the contractions start.' And that helps make you feel a bit better, that you're not totally defenseless."

More than any issue concerning the birth process, Elena remembered the midwife's assertions that patients should know about their treatment and their autonomy vis-à-vis the health care institution. Yet she had also heard numerous rumors that led her to feel wary about the anonymous doctors she was about to encounter in the hospital. "I've heard that sometimes, when they don't want to keep women in the maternity home for a long time, they give them shots, like on a conveyer belt, you know, to get them out." Elena spoke in a matter-of-fact tone, suggesting that it seemed entirely plausible to her that the hospital could routinely give all women injections to stimulate labor, for the sole purpose of the staff's own convenience. She had no trust that the institution itself was bound by a series of ethics and a commitment to treating each woman as an individual.

Still, the prenatal midwife advised arriving at the hospital prior to the start of labor, "as a precaution." Having had a healthy pregnancy without complications and having a history of no abortions, health problems, or previous pregnancies, Elena considered herself healthy. She decided to admit herself to the hospital in the days before labor merely as a safety precaution, as a way of acting responsibly: "All my analyses were normal. The women's consultation center just suggested that I come early, and I figured that I'd insure myself. It's the first baby, and I want to be careful. If you wait to the last minute, who knows what will happen."

At the same time, Elena remained anxious about the doctors' trustworthiness and planned to make every effort to understand their procedures and prescriptions. Her first encounters with the staff increased that unease. She described her experiences when she came to the hospital for information about their admitting procedures:

I came here the eighth of May [to be admitted]. I came here during the week before [also] in order to find out information about being admitted, [such as] when to come, what to bring, all these kinds of questions. But they [at the admitting desk] didn't let us in. They [originally had] told us we could come for a consultation [with the doctors], but then [when we arrived] at the [information] door, they said rudely, "What do you need to know? I'll tell you!" I came with my friend who's also going to give birth soon. It's truly a bit cruel.

Although the hospital had a policy of free public consultations with physicians, Elena was refused entry with no explanation, confirming her fears about the dominance of the institution and the insignificance of individual patients' needs. And a few days later, Elena experienced the brunt of the behavior she knew as characteristic of "our system."

To pursue the matter of physician-patient interactions, I asked Elena how Nina Petrovna acted toward her following the outburst the day before.

"This morning she came around on the rounds and was a bit nicer. I've heard that she's an excellent specialist. But this whole thing has shocked me. I thought that in a maternity home it would be different, not like this. When someone's about to give birth, you can't yell at them, just as you can't yell at a sick person. And it affects the baby too. I told my friend, she's due in a few weeks, don't come here. My roommate wants to leave now, to be discharged and go to a maternity home where you can pay. . . . I've been here since the eighth of May and I feel like I've been here a year. I should give birth on the eleventh or twelfth; they explained to me that the shots will help make the birth come faster and the tablets I take should take away the swelling."

Elena's account reveals the sense of vulnerability shared by many women who confronted public health care institutions. The matter-of-fact tone in which Elena told me that maternity homes were reputed to "give women shots, like on a conveyer belt . . . to get them out" suggests that the rumors she has heard seemed entirely realistic to her. If the advice she received from the prenatal clinic's midwife, that "you have the right to refuse and to sign a document that says you want to leave" initially seemed reassuring, it was in actuality quite vague information. Elena did not know the name of the document, had no insights into how to demand this "right," and was not warned about the psychological pressures providers would use to enforce her compliance. From her account of the midwife's lectures, in fact, they promoted proper patient behavior and respect for expert authority, rather than women's individual empowerment. "She told us what symptoms you have and how to behave. She told us the names of medicines since doctors want you to know them," Elena recalled. And with no concrete sense of systemic protections and specific procedures to take for protecting herself, her fear of doctors as an anonymous mass of agents of the state, empowered without restraint, persisted. She was left with only individualized means of protection.

Elena and other women considered themselves to be taking responsibility for their health precisely by maintaining distrust in the official medical system. By reading medical textbooks on their own, avoiding health care institutions to the greatest extent possible, and insisting that they learn the details of their treatment despite the hostile reproaches of providers, they actively coped with the sense that the hospital was a source of immanent danger: a site of infection, or a factory-like atmosphere run by indifferent, self-interested providers who at best took unnecessary steps to "over-insure" themselves at the expense of women's well-being, and at worst induced harm by giving injections to lighten their own work load. By withholding trust from their providers, these patients saw themselves struggling against the personal embodiments of "our system."

Women's reluctance to endow physicians with authority on the basis of their expert status alone suggests an important way that local knowledge of state power differed under socialist and capitalist conditions. Bourdieu, for example, was struck by the readiness of laypersons to attribute authority to professionals in France, and explained this trust as the routine misrecognition of state power (1994). When patients take the provider's license as a sign of her individual talent and skill, they implicitly accept the legitimacy of the state as arbitrating agent of expertise and responsibility. The state-issued license serves the professional as a "certificate of charisma," transforming the person into a bona fide healer (Bourdieu 1990: 138; 1994: 11–12). Bourdieu developed this analysis to highlight that the license, first and foremost, attests to a physician's compliance with the state bureaucracy, with its arguably random or at least partial criteria of expert standards; and he urged laypersons to recognize that ceding authority to a person merely because she is endowed by the state with a "certificate of charisma" serves primarily to naturalize and reproduce conditions of inequality. In the Russian context, as we have seen, the situation was quite the reverse. Patients anticipated that doctors were likely to be "indifferent" [*ravnodushno, bezrazlichno*] to patient needs and to seek all possible means of escaping responsibility for their work. These traits, importantly, were directly related to providers' association with the official health care system, itself considered to be a microcosm of "our system"—the delegitimized, collapsed, but still influential Soviet bureaucracy. Turning Bourdieu's concept around, we can say that in the eyes of many Russian patients, doctors' licenses as medical experts—as all evidence of their association with the state—not only failed to generate trust but actually raised disturbing suspicions that they would replicate negative practices associated with the state system. Their licenses from the state constituted certificates without charisma.

PROVIDERS' STRATEGIES

On a daily basis and in almost ritual fashion, providers told stories about the poor treatment they received from hospital administrators and patients. Despite the division of patient care into distinct wards with separate staffs, nothing prevented the hospital grapevine from flowing freely to all employees, of all ranks. Lively oral narratives transformed the sting of personal humiliation into a shared experience, creating a sense of unity and camaraderie. These stories created and reaffirmed an organization of the world as divided between "us" medical workers and "them"—a depersonalized other who in one case might consist of patients and in another, administrators. The stories served to socialize new hospital employees to express a proper allegiance with other employees and to disassociate themselves from any group potentially categorized as other. They also revealed those rewards that providers most coveted but experienced as most elusive: respect, deference, authority.

Stories about the administration were the most bitter, because the administration was perceived as the direct source of providers' subordination. On several occasions, Natalia Borisovna invited friends of hers to come to the hospital after work to provide services to staff: once a former patient volunteered to organize aerobics classes for anyone interested; another time the husband of a former patient offered his hairdressing services. These events boosted morale and helped compensate for providers' low salaries, for they were provided either free or at rates substantially lower than one could obtain commercially. In both cases, the administration refused permission. "I've already had my hair cut," the hospital's second-in-command self-righteously retorted when Natalia Borisovna approached her with the idea. Symbolic slaps in the face such as this, emphasizing providers' limited scope for independence, surpassed mere inconsiderateness. Physicians felt abused on a daily basis. "Nelly Ivanovna [the hospital's chief doctor] yells at us everyday. If I'm the first one from the floor she sees, she'll yell at me, because I'm convenient. She'll yell at any of us. Every morning at the staff meeting we get yelled at. It happens all day, every day, all the time," Nina Petrovna told me.

Over the course of twelve months of fieldwork in this hospital, I learned that almost all its staff felt alienated and under attack by their hospital's administrators. Nelly Ivanovna maintained a stern, inflexible manner with her subordinates in order to create strict discipline among the staff. Most work-related decisions were made unilaterally, and the staff was consequently informed that new policies such as rotating schedules would be implemented. Following a tragic case of a patient's death, Nelly Ivanovna informed Natalia Borisovna that she would be representing the hospital's side of the story to the city's Public Health Committee, despite her total lack of involvement in the case. There were no choices, no negotiations possible with this administration. Physicians often clammed up and grew silent when hospital administrators came to their floor; when administrators phoned physicians to convey an order, the conversations were formal, brief, and cold. It was not uncommon for physicians even with extensive work tenure to be berated by administrators in front of patients.

Karina told me another story exemplifying the frustrating, humiliating experience of vertical hierarchy. The maternity hospital's heating supply, like that in all institutional and residential buildings in the city, was controlled by a centralized city center. One day, in the middle of November, the heat was suddenly and noticeably lowered. Women were cold and began asking to bring in radiators from home to heat their rooms. The word from the administrators' office was that nobody should bring in anything. Yet there was no direct communication from Nelly Ivanovna, no formal announcement, just a shake of the head from her secretary. In the morning of the next day, Natalia Borisovna went to Nelly Ivanovna and asked permission for women to bring in radiators. Approaching the chief doctor was always an emotionally fraught experience, and this time was no different. Nelly Ivanovna announced her refusal, gave no explanation, did not discuss the issue, and dismissed the prenatal ward chief. Another day went by, and the women were cold, the providers were cold. The next day an accident occurred at the central heating source in the region and the heat was turned off altogether. Karina told me what happened that morning:

> The hospital was cold as a freezer, and we had to tell these relatives who are coming to take care of their pregnant wives, daughters, sisters, "No, you can't bring in radiators." Then by the afternoon finally word comes through that it's OK to do so. And we're asking the women to figure out who lives the closest and has a radiator at home with relatives to bring it over. Finally, we call the relatives and ask them to come with it. It was such a miserable experience, we all felt so powerless. It was an absurd situation and it just killed us to feel so impotent.

Stories about patients and their families targeted a broader range of behaviors, although defiance and aggressiveness were traits considered most infuriating. One story involved a highly esteemed physician, Mikhail Vinogradov, who had recently completed a Ph.D. and was on his way to becoming one of the city's top medical researchers as well as practitioners. Hospital staff universally regarded this doctor highly for his research, his self-assured, meticulous professionalism, and his ironic wit. Because he was one of the few male staff members, they treated him affectionately and nicknamed him Vinograd (grapes). A story told about an encounter Vinograd had with the relatives of one patient was narrated time and time again among staff, and captured the demeaning behavior that could result when patients mistrusted physicians and felt unrestrained by the laws of civility in attempts to get their due. The story goes that one afternoon Vinograd met with a patient's husband and mother-in-law to tell them that their relative was not well enough to be discharged, despite the fact that it was the fifth day since the birth, the usual day for discharges. Before he had a chance to explain the nature of the complications and his treatment plan, the relatives pounced on him, reproaching him for his incompetence. Instead of expressing worries or concern, the relatives admonished Vinograd for not fulfilling his obligations. "It's your job to make sure she's healthy; you're supposed to be knowledgeable and capable, and obviously you're not," they blared. This attitude, Karina explained, was common: patients confronted physicians with an unrelenting blend of dissatisfaction, blame, and entitlement, conveying through their words and actions the message "you're incompetent, and you owe me."

Another story spread through the maternity hospital and was told and retold by staff with nothing less than glee. One doctor, Svetlana Grigoreevna, was in the delivery room with a woman in the early stages of labor. Not realizing Svetlana Grigoreevna was a physician, the woman asked her to bring the bedpan. Svetlana Grigoreevna told the woman that she was still able to get up and walk, and therefore should use the bathroom. The woman turned to the health care worker and announced, "I'll pay you." Shocked and insulted, Svetlana Grigoreevna retorted, "You don't have enough money!" Providers loved this tale because it performed a symbolic victory over patients who seemed to parade their money around as if it held the key to the world. While doctors saw their deserved status and rights to just compensation repeatedly betrayed, this story showed they could nonetheless "win back" a sense of hierarchy rhetorically, by asserting their high value and superiority over patients directly to them: "*You* could never afford to pay *me*."

The bitter flavor of these stories left me feeling cold and awkward, unwilling to appreciate the humor in these reciprocal but uneven humiliations. Getting to know the providers helped me understand—if not excuse—their resentment of patients, as pained expressions of the collapse of lifelong dreams. Most physicians I met at No. 5 and elsewhere in Russia had entered medicine soon after high school as devoted idealists, filled with an intense sense of duty and obligation to heal others. There was no possibility of lucrative compensation. Students entered medical institutes aware that they would face a lifetime of longer work hours and lower wages than their less educated neighbors working in factories. Yet time and again I heard doctors explain that outside of medicine, "there was simply nothing else I could do with my life." Natalia Borisovna described obstetrics as the second most important thing a person could do in this world, diminished only by the contribution of soldiers who had defended the homeland during World War II. "I couldn't be part of that group," she explained, "so I decided to deliver babies." If the expected reward was not monetary, it was supposed to be of an even higher order in the collective society—social admiration and authority. Recalling her favorite Chekhov stories, Natalia Borisovna nostalgically described how *zemskii* doctors in pre-revolutionary Russia enjoyed immense respect from their communities. The Soviet system, however, had ruined their status and sown the seeds of patient distrust, she explained. Instead of a family doctor with holistic training embedded in the community he treated, the Soviet system had fragmented medical expertise and care into isolated, atomistic units. The result was fatal, she claimed, for it made it exceedingly difficult to be fully competent as a healer. "We obstetricians have to do everything ourselves," she griped, lamenting the lack of support from other specialists. While required to know about all possible kinds of non-gynecological illnesses that may complicate a pregnancy, obstetricians had neither the training nor the structure of services to ensure this knowledge:

> They tell us things, the eye doctors, the cardiologists, the venereal disease specialists, but we must know as much as they do, because we have to make the decisions ourselves. They don't want to take responsibility for these problems. . . . The gynecologists at the prenatal clinic just write everything down and give the patient her records. She brings it to us, and we have to decide what to do with it all.

When I asked whether she and other physicians investigated patients' cases by contacting caregivers from other institutions, Natalia Borisovna quickly asserted that this was an impossible burden to assume. She then redirected the conversation to challenge my assumption that obstetricians should or could be responsible for women's health: "No, first of all, we can't. They're all over the city and we don't have time to do that. The women think that the doctors must take care of their pregnancies. They don't take care of themselves. In your country, every woman must take care of herself. Our system has told women, you know better than doctors. For seventy years, they said, 'Doctors are stupid.'"

When I looked at her quizzically, she continued sarcastically with an example:

> Read that wonderful magazine, *Zdorov'e*.[5] These are very bad from the doctor's point of view. We think women should go to the doctor, but she reads these books, and she gets illegal medicine without a prescription, and she performs all sorts of treatments herself, or she'll go to the doctor but she won't take the medicine. The doctor

studies ten years and should know what medicine a woman should take. But the woman thinks that she knows better than the doctor. She has no trust in doctors.

As I listened to this heaping pile of grievances, my head spun. No one else took responsibility for women's health, Natalia Borisovna complained: prenatal gynecologists and other medical specialists shirked responsibility for pregnant women, passing the buck to obstetricians. Women patients failed to care for themselves, yet expected doctors "to take care of their pregnancies," and then, not trusting doctors, failed to comply with experts' instructions. This logic made it clear that women could not win: if they turned toward the health provider with anticipations of assistance, they were berated for "not taking care of themselves," but if they attempted to inform themselves on issues related to their own health, women were accused of showing disrespect toward medical expertise. Natalia Borisovna saw all of these problems as rooted in "our system," which she blamed for both creating the impossible division of labor and urging patients' lack of compliance. Her frustration with the larger public health system and patient attitudes was exacerbated by the inflexible, authoritarian management style of her hospital administration. With no leeway to determine her own work schedule or negotiate changes in her position to suit her personal and family needs, Natalia Borisovna felt that her job—her calling in life—had been transformed into a source of endless disappointment and frustration, with blows from all sides, and little sign of the appreciation and respect she knew to be her due.

There were three ways providers could cope with the collective irresponsibility structured into the public health system, Karina explained to me. There were those who exploited the system and benefited from it; those who accepted it and did their best within it while swallowing its inadequacies and lowering their expectations; and those who fought it. Doctors who fought it struggled against this system because they felt called to medicine and were motivated by deep concerns to alleviate human suffering and ensure people's health. Natalia Borisovna earned the highest respect from her colleagues because of her total devotion to her work. She followed up on her patients' deliveries despite having no official part in most of their births and postpartum care. Each night that she was not on duty in the delivery room, she walked her dog past the hospital to see which patients' lights were on and whether there was activity in the delivery room. Through her actions no less than her words, this obstetrician consistently demonstrated that she would fulfill her obligations with the highest caliber medical care. At times these qualities could be seen as threatening by other providers, who resented such high standards, which they did not feel able or willing to meet. After Natalia Borisovna resigned, she was replaced by an obstetrician who was new to the hospital, but who had already heard of her predecessor's reputation. "I'm not Natalia Borisovna," Ekaterina Aleksandrovna immediately warned her new colleagues. "I can't work like she worked, and you shouldn't expect the same things from me. I'll do what I can." And in Karina's view, Ekaterina Aleksandrovna knew herself well. Once, a woman in her thirty-fifth week of pregnancy felt sharp pains in her stomach area, but tests revealed there were no contractions. Ekaterina Aleksandrovna suspected appendicitis, told the patient, and called for a specialist. After some time had passed and nobody attended her, the woman pressed the doctor for an update. "Why do you keep bothering me?" Ekaterina Aleksandrovna barked back. "Can't you see I've just come off a twenty-four-hour shift? I'm exhausted and need to finish writing my case histories. I already called the specialist; he'll come when he comes!" The response shocked Karina, who said that Natalia Borisovna would never have spoken to a woman this way. "What would she have said?" I asked, having heard Natalia Borisovna use an exasperated tone with frightened women more than once. "She would've said, "I'm in charge and I'm taking care of everything. You need to take hold of yourself and think about the health of your child. Worrying will not help. Everything is under control." The difference between the two did not consist of degrees of gentleness and closeness, as I initially expected, but of the ways the doctors accepted responsibility for the patient's situation. Natalia Borisovna, Karina explained, would remind the patient that the doctor was in control of the situation. She would never unload her own problems, such as being tired or overburdened, on a patient. She never sought to escape from responsibility.

Another part of this commitment involved forging supportive relations among staff, boosting morale, and ensuring the hospital's best possible performance with patients. But with an administration bent on destroying any initiatives from below, as Natalia Borisovna had attempted in organizing after-work events, taking responsibility was a constant struggle. Involving oneself in matters where one wasn't obliged or invited, Karina explained, resulted in a predictable response from "our system," known as "the streetcar law": if you stick your neck out, it'll get cut off. Don't intervene, don't interfere, stay in your place and everything will go smoothly. Natalia Borisovna, Nina Petrovna, and Vinograd saw themselves struggling against a system that generated allegiance to the vertical hierarchy and supported the system of collective irresponsibility. They belonged to the third category, Karina explained, and earned the respect of their colleagues. But they also suffered tremendously, a price paid through increasing cynicism, resentment, and bitterness. As we saw with the case of Elena above, these committed doctors were not immune from deploying "the streetcar law" themselves as they strove to take responsibility for their work and ensure healthy childbearing for their patients.

INDIVIDUALIZED SOLUTIONS

When providers and patients used the concept of "our system" to capture the palpable dimensions of state power, they recognized the obstacles to healthy reproduction, such as fragmented services, incompetent care, and widespread indifference, as *collective* kinds of constraints. Yet both groups dealt with these obstacles through individualized or personalized tactics. Collective forms of action, such as developing health users' lobbying or support groups, or health workers' associations, were outside everyone's imaginative possibilities. Instead, they prided themselves on taking personal responsibility for improving health and, when possible, individually demanding responsibility from the other. While many accounts of life in Russia have suggested that investing in the self and interpersonal relations offered people an important means of coping with the unsatisfactory systems of daily life under state socialism, these practices in the public maternity hospital show that a moral focus on personhood as opposed to politics continued in the mid 1990s.

At the same time, this was not a clear-cut story of "morality" against a tainted realm of officialdom. Doctors disassociated themselves from the state in selective ways, mainly by rejecting those facets of "our system" they felt victimized by. Sometimes they forged intimate circles of trust as emotional buffers against the harsh, insensitive administrators above. At other times providers tried to disassociate themselves from "our system" by attacking women patients, who were the most vulnerable group in this state sphere but whom providers often regarded as perpetrators of "our system" in its apathy about health and insolence toward expertise. Such symbolic disassociations from "our system," combined with providers' efforts to increase their authority as medical experts, thus involved ignoring their own entanglement in state power. Doctors were simultaneously victimized and empowered by the state bureaucracy; they both tried to resist it and successfully reproduced it. And sadly, these coping strategies inadvertently facilitated the state's abandonment of public health by turning resistance inward toward the clinic, rather than outward toward the public sphere.

Patients such as Elena similarly complicate assumptions that people under socialism rejected any involvement in practices associated with the "official" realm of the state. While rumors and personal experiences raised Elena's suspicions about the kind of care she might encounter in the maternity hospital, she nonetheless expected humane, sensitive treatment. She both met with the worst displays of hostility she knew as typical of "our system" and also found a prenatal midwife she trusted and a hospital nurse who treated her well. Elena struggled to protect herself against the abuses possible at the hands of "our system," but also agreed to admit herself to the maternity hospital before labor began "as a precaution," suggesting that while she remained guarded about the safety and competence of the state institution, she did not totally distrust it. In her view, "our system" constituted the harmful, aggressive, destructive aspects of state power, a force that emanated from structures and systems but worked its violence through the employees it inhabited. Her efforts to ensure a safe birth centered on becoming personally empowered to understand the procedures and to stand up to the recalcitrant representatives of "our system" whom she unfortunately encountered.

Who represented "our system" shifted endlessly in providers' and patients' discourses. This common sense logic of locating injustice at the site of abusive forms of state power, rather than in a single group, helps explain why a shared, static identity such as gender did not become a basis for solidarity and activism. Women patients and providers did not see power and vulnerability as neatly mapping onto one group or another against which they could unify and struggle. Any individual might experience multiple layers of power and subordination, and these emerged or became submerged at different moments of time. The case of a physician in the postnatal ward who shared lunches and informal camaraderie with Natalia Borisovna and Nina Petrovna for years before accepting a high administrative post in the hospital illustrates this further. Once she became an administrator, this doctor cut off friendly interactions with her new subordinates and reproduced the disciplinary tactics she had previously critiqued. When I expressed shock and dismay, Natalia Borisovna simply explained, "Power changes people. It can't be any other way" (cf. Pesmen 2000). On the other hand, despite doctors' animosity toward women en masse, they knew that patients, too, suffered from numerous problems and vulnerabilities within and outside the health sphere. Two final stories of institutional mistrust and personal connection illustrate this, and shed light on the ways solidarity between providers and patients sometimes emerged.

Soon after meeting Natalia Borisovna, I also became acquainted with her friend Nadia. Nadia frequently met Natalia Borisovna after work and several times a week went home with her former doctor to eat dinner and help take care of Natalia Borisovna's two children. When the physicians in the maternity home got together to celebrate a colleague's birthday or attend the theater, Nadia usually accompanied Natalia Borisovna. The circumstances under which their relationship was forged, however, were characterized by an alienation and lack of trust in "our system" that far surpassed any interaction I witnessed during my fieldwork. Two years earlier, when Nadia was thirty weeks pregnant, she had been admitted to the gynecological unit of the maternity hospital with an emergency case of eclampsia. A single twenty-six-year-old woman who had no relationship with the father of her expected baby and no close friends, Nadia had as her sole "support" her mother, an abusive woman whom Nadia avoided as much as possible. Despite this conflictual relationship, Nadia took her mother's advice to regard the hospital staff with great suspicion and not take any medications the physicians prescribed. As Nadia told me, during the entire week she was on the ward, she threw the pills Natalia Borisovna prescribed out of her hospital room window, convinced that they were harmful. "My mother kept telling me that they give everyone the same pills, without even noticing who you are, or what you need," Nadia explained. "And I believed her. I didn't know Natalia Borisovna, and I couldn't imagine how much she cares about her patients. She really suffers for them," Nadia said.

In the course of the week, Nadia's complications continued to worsen, and in the seventh month of gestation, the baby died. Alone, deeply depressed, and unable to confront her mother, Nadia turned to Natalia Borisovna for comfort. They had been virtually inseparable ever since. Nadia told me that Natalia Borisovna was, to that day, consumed with guilt that she had not been able to convince Nadia to trust her and take the prescribed medicine. "She can't forgive herself," Nadia told me. "But nothing would have changed my mind," she added.

I considered this relationship to be quite exceptional for the first five months of my fieldwork in maternity home no. 5. But something then happened that made me question the infrequency of such physician-provider friendships. When I returned to the field after a brief absence due to health problems, Nina Petrovna was talking incessantly about someone whom I had never heard of before, a woman named Sasha. Sasha had a car (a luxury none of the doctors had), and she was coming to the maternity hospital every day at the end of Nina Petrovna's shift to pick her up. They were enjoying regular weekend trips to the parks surrounding St. Petersburg and the countryside, and even planning a summer vacation by car to the Crimea. When I finally inquired who Sasha was, Nina Petrovna sighed and said, "I'll tell you the story." She then explained that while I was gone, Sasha, a single thirty-year-old woman then in her eighth month of pregnancy, was brought to the hospital in an ambulance for urgent treatment. Her mother, outraged at Sasha's intent to bear a child out of wedlock, had kicked her in the stomach. Nina Petrovna found internal bleeding and delivered the baby by emergency c-section, but it did not live. For days, Sasha cried inconsolably in the maternity home. As her physical recovery progressed, she told Nina Petrovna the details of her life. It was clear to both of them that Sasha could not return to her mother's house, but she had nowhere else to go. The father of her baby was married to someone else, and Sasha had no friends who could take her in with them. Nina Petrovna, after consulting with her adult daughter, Marina, invited Sasha to stay with them until she got her life arranged anew. At the time Nina Petrovna told me this story, Sasha had been living with Nina Petrovna and Marina in their two-room apartment for over six weeks, and the physician did not foresee anything changing in the near future. Though their relationship was not free from conflict (Sasha's drinking was a constant concern to Nina Petrovna), they had become close friends. Like Natalia Borisovna and Nadia, they had formed a relationship based on trust, even a kind of kinship, as they called each other *svoi* [one's own]. The sympathy and mutual caregiving that shaped these bonds held all the characteristics of relationships I had often seen between Russian women—such as practical support at home, communicative warmth, and active nurturance. But they did not involve a consciousness of gendered oppression and interests. Indeed, Nadia and Sasha spoke of their doctor-friends' devotion to medicine, their brilliance as experts, and their frustrating situations at work. Yet they never equated their own experiences of suffering with those of their doctors; a doctor's womanhood was considered a totally irrelevant matter.

FIVE

Personal Ties and the Authorization of Medical Power

The afternoon Nina Petrovna told me the story of her new friend, Sasha, we were strolling through St. Petersburg's downtown stalls of street vendors, enjoying some time away from the stresses of the maternity hospital. After hearing this moving account of how she reached out to a patient in desperate need, I mentioned to her that I was interested in the ethics of provider-patient relations, and asked what she thought of this issue. Nina Petrovna answered me frankly that she consciously acted "cold" to her patients, both in order to get her large amount of work done and to avoid appearing to play favorites:

> You know, I don't want to get close to the women. I purposefully maintain distance from them. I'm sure they've told you that they don't like me, that I'm rigid and stern with them. The thing is, I don't have much time. I have to see each patient, and if I was to talk with each of them, I'd never get it all done. I spend most of my time as it is doing nonmedical work, writing paperwork. If I had a computer and a Dicta-phone, and a secretary to do the paperwork for me, I'd be able to do other things perhaps. . . . The thing is that if I talk with one or two, then the other patients think that I'm getting money for this, and that's why I'm treating them better. I hold them all at a distance. You know, sometimes you like someone a bit better and you'll talk a bit with them, but in general, I am cold to them. I do this purposefully, I'm cold to them on purpose.

"Well, what do you say, for example, when your daughter Marina or one of your friends visits a doctor who acts cold? What do you think of that?" I asked.

At first, Nina Petrovna argued that medical skills were the most important issue in health care, while the bedside manner was rather negligible.

"You can be a good doctor, do everything well professionally, and just say, 'yes, yes, yes,' and that's all. I'd rather have a doctor like that than someone who says, 'Oh, my love, how are you dear,' and is very affectionate, but doesn't do a thing medically."

"But what do you say to Marina or one of your friends when they come into contact with a doctor who is cold?" I pressed her.

"For the most part we all see each other, we get checked out by each other. Marina too, so that's all she really knows. When she learned that we act this way formally, she was shocked. She couldn't believe it."

An important cultural distinction emerged in this discussion, one crucial for making sense of the informal, personalizing strategies that providers and patients undertook in the 1990s to improve women's health care. One the one hand, Nina Petrovna expressed concern that any privileged treatment she showed to some patients would be interpreted as a sign that she was profiting materially by accepting illicit payments from women. In the mid 1990s, taking money from patients was strictly taboo at this hospital, a policy rigidly enforced by the chief doctor and normatively accepted by all the staff providers I had come to know. On the other hand, Nina Petrovna discussed other informal practices as quite common: the tendency for people with connections in the medical field to be treated by acquaintances and for medical professionals to treat their acquaintances quite differently, indeed, with the warmth one would want shown to one's own daughter.

Acquaintance relations [*znakomstvo, blat*] are used as strategies for improving women's health care and overcoming the constraining dimensions of "our system." Much ink has been spilled in analyses of socialism that discuss the importance of informal connections for daily survival. Usually these relations are described as strategies for obtaining goods in short supply or for expediting bureaucratic services. Scholars have recently drawn attention to the explicitly moral character of many informal exchanges, to rectify visions of the "second economy" as wholly utilitarian, and a key to the presumed anomie of life under socialism (Ledeneva 1998; Pesmen 2000).[1] Ledeneva's study of *blat* under socialism showed how Russia's "economy of favors" both overlapped with and differed from Western practices of corruption and bribery. If *blat* relations countered formal laws to establish an unofficial redistribution of privilege, they nonetheless differed from bribery in significant ways: *blat* relations aimed to fulfill needs that the state promised but failed to ensure; they were related to altruism; and they were motivated by a moral obligation to help out kin and friends in situations of want (1998: 39–42). Ledeneva distinguishes between different regimes of reciprocity that shaped the vast array of informal relations in daily life. Two modes of exchange relations are particularly useful for our purposes: regimes of equivalence and regimes of affection. Regimes of equivalence were marked by an expectation that the relationship could have potential mutual "utility." Even here, notably, people did not calculate a balance of favors or weigh the objects exchanged—rather, it was the quality of the relationship that partners appraised. A second type of relationship was governed by the "regime of affection." In such relationships, personal ties preceded a given *blat* encounter. Moments of assistance, consequently, were marked by compatible "standards of value, mutual sympathy and satisfaction" (Ledeneva 1998: 144–48). In other words, participants in these relations shared a mutual concern for the other's well-being that drove them to initiate offers of assistance, as one of Ledeneva's informants stated: "It is important to be useful to the other, in other words, *to care*" (1998: 148; emphasis added).

Obtaining maternity services per se was not an issue for any pregnant woman in St. Petersburg in the mid 1990s, for immediate, free care was assured and, before 1998, deficits in necessary medications were minimal. Rather than seeking to obtain basic supplies or cut through red tape, Russians formed acquaintance networks in medical care for more intangible goals: to ensure competent attention and committed care. Patients sought to transcend the bureaucratic framework of doctor-patient relations that worked on the basis of anonymity and fragmented care by personalizing it, transforming the health care setting into an extension of one's personal relations. Physicians found through acquaintance chains were perceived as "trustworthy" not because their medical skills were reputed to be better, but because they were expected to care for a patient-acquaintance out of *personal* concern, *rather than* bureaucratic obligation.

Doctors, however, intuitively distinguished between the kinds of personal relations and appeals for special attention that patients confronted them with, and responded in dramatically different ways to presentations under the regime of equivalence and the regime of affection. Inasmuch as the regime of equivalence displayed a more overtly utilitarian character, it often failed to generate provider sympathy. Doctors resented acquaintances who offered them bribes in return for special treatment because such suggestions revealed the patients' lack of trust in the providers' integrity and commitment to all patients. Rather than expensive "gifts" or money, doctors sought symbolic recognition of their authority through signs of patient trust and sincere gratitude. (Material gifts given in the appropriate manner, consequently, could be accepted if they conveyed such intangible meanings.) Thus, doctors gladly provided extra attention to women acquaintances who greeted them with expressions of thanks and appreciation—in Ledeneva's terms, with whom they shared "standards of value." The regime of affection, unlike the regime of equivalence, symbolically removed the doctor-patient relation from the framework of the bureau-cratic state system into a morally compelling framework of personal obli-gation.

As an example of daily strategies for overcoming the bonds of socialist constraint ("our system"), acquaintance relations under the regime of af-fection reveal the profound emotional dimension that often accompanied personalizing activities: treating one's relative or friend with care and con-cern felt right, decent, necessary. Relying on the close-knit circle of health care providers considered *svoi* [one of us] enabled Nina Petrovna and vir-tually all medical professionals to shield themselves and their families from the bureaucratic constraints of health care delivered in the framework of "our system" and the harsh treatment often associated with it. Personal re-lations also enabled providers to misrecognize that they themselves enact-ed the sociability of "our system." Nina Petrovna could justify her "cold" attitude toward patients as a necessity given her difficult work conditions, maintain the conviction that she effectively fulfilled her obligations as a medical professional, and extend her informal circle of social protection to include her closest kin and friends when they became patients. In this way, personalizing strategies in the health care realm reproduced the distinction between "us"—the ordinary, suffering people—and "them"—the power-ful—found in many contexts under socialism (Gal and Kligman 2000a: 51–52). The profoundly mobilizing sensibility that oriented people to take care of those considered "one of *us*," moreover, marginalized the impor-tance of a shared gender identity between providers and patients. It en-sured that the forms of solidarity they did create would be based on identi-ties that were personal and informal, rather than collective and social.

The use of acquaintance relations to ensure trust in provider-patient relations also offers insights into how Russian women negotiated expert dominance and attributed authority to physicians' medical knowledge. Women sought to mobilize acquaintance relations to ensure providers' personal concern and commitment, their willingness to assume responsi-bility. Women did not conceptualize their needs through a language of "self-determination" and "rights," as WHO suggested. Indeed, the Rus-sian-English translator at WHO's workshop, a St. Petersburg native with perfect English, told me that she rejected the agency's model of contra-ceptive counseling based on provider "neutrality" and patient "empower-ment." I traveled home with Anya after the workshop ended, and she adamantly insisted, "I wouldn't want a doctor to tell me about the range of contraceptives available, list the pros and cons of each, and leave it to me to decide alone. I'd like them to say, 'I'd advise you to use this one.' That would show they care. Anya confirmed that trust in providers and willing-ness to attribute authority to their medical knowledge were based at least partly in the form of the social relationship she had with them. By displaying emotional involvement and personal commitment in a patients' care, providers relieved women's suspicions that they were indifferent and avoided taking responsibility for their work. Displays of care and commitment by acquaintances often formed the basis for women's judgments of medical power as legitimate. While this process is clearly linked to the specific logic of constraints under state socialism, I believe it holds relevance to broader feminist inquiries of medicalization. To understand whether medical dominance becomes legitimate and what forms biomedical power takes, we must examine the institutional context and social relations framing provider-patient relations (Lazarus 1990; Lock and Kaufert 1998).

SONIA'S STORY: PERSONALIZING THE BUREAUCRACY, AUTHORIZING MEDICAL POWER

As a service to the community, maternity hospital No. 5 initiated weekly outpatient consultations, where pregnant women could meet individually with a staff obstetrician. Similar meetings were being arranged by maternity hospitals establishing paid services, so that patients willing to buy fee-for-service care would have a chance to learn about the new procedures and "extra" services they could now access. At maternity hospital No. 5, there was no fee-for-service childbirth. Still, the administration recognized that with prenatal care structurally separate, such consultations would offer a valuable opportunity for women to get a sense of the hospital and learn about its admitting process. Frequently, women learned of the consultations through acquaintances of the staff themselves, for there was no advertising or "outreach" to neighborhood residents. Nonetheless, word traveled fast, and twice a week in the afternoons, the obstetricians met with prospective patients who were mostly in their third trimesters. One such consultation I attended with Natalia Borisovna in the spring of 1995 offered me dramatic insights into the informal strategies that patients and providers deployed, under still extant socialist conditions,[2] for pursuing competent care and achieving healthy reproductive outcomes.

When Natalia Borisovna entered the outpatient consultation room this particular afternoon, she greeted Sonia with a comfortable smile, almost as if meeting an old friend. As they began reviewing her medical chart, Natalia Borisovna created a warm, trusting atmosphere by speaking to Sonia gently, addressing her alternately with the affectionate diminutive "Soniachka" and the even more familiar "my child." Combined with the gentleness of her tone, these endearments made Natalia Borisovna's use of the familiar form of "you" [ty] seem friendly, rather than a demeaning marker of subordination. Her voice was caring, but unmistakably cautious. In fact, Natalia Borisovna's concern for Sonia far surpassed the level of attention usually shown a woman with a healthy pregnancy, and I soon realized that Sonia's was not a routine pregnancy.

Natalia Borisovna began by inquiring, "How are you feeling?"

"Ok, it's moving OK, I feel OK. My first baby's head also was up here, and it's feet down there. He'll probably turn around."

Natalia Borisovna checked Sonia's chart and then asked, "How many weeks do you think you are—thirty-six?"

"Yes, I think so. I had two ultrasounds, the first at nineteen weeks."

"So you had an abortion in 1990 and in '91 a miscarriage?"

"Yes, at twelve weeks, I came in bleeding. The first pregnancy was born [but] it was a breech. The birth, counting from the start of contractions, lasted eighteen hours. He was alive when born, then the doctor came to resuscitate him and said that due to the head trauma, he died."

"Oh, my dear child, I understand everything [*moia detka vse poniatno*]."

Natalia Borisovna continued, noting Sonia's low hemoglobin and high blood pressure, and then recommended that Sonia be admitted for rest and observation. "Soniachka, I want to tell you that you should probably stay here for about ten days. All the signs indicate that you'll have a c-section; you're thirty years old, have no baby yet, [but] maybe you'll give birth yourself [vaginally]."

"Are there any exercises to turn the baby around?"

"No. At thirty-eight weeks we'll have to decide together what to do. You have to be here then, we have to give you a baby. There's no question about this, you must rest, get off your feet."

Feeling the top of Sonia's uterus, she confirmed the breech position. "I feel the head is lying here." She then changed the subject, "You can stay home or we could admit you now; we should decide."

Sonia was not eager to be admitted, and asked, "Can I walk around in the park?"

"It's better to sit on the bench, walk a bit and bend over a bit. Do you wash the floor?"

"Yes."

"So that's enough exercise. I'll write you the prescription for the pills you need, Trentol or [unclear], it's the same group; take them three times a week, take Vitamin E for fourteen days, definitely take iron. Also, if you can take [unclear] do it, twice a day for fourteen days, and I'll wait for you at thirty-eight weeks. Do you understand? And tell them at the prenatal clinic that you came for a consultation at the maternity hospital where you gave birth the first time."

"At the prenatal clinic the doctor told me not to worry."

"Worry. Be careful, don't run around."

"I know, if I feel bad I have to take it easy and I won't refuse being admitted [to the maternity hospital]."

Natalia Borisovna then looked at Sonia seriously, and with an urgent but caring tone said, "Listen, I'm asking you, Soniachka, if your head or your stomach hurts, please call and tell me, and come right over. We may need to admit you for observation. This is very important, we need to get you this baby. Be careful, don't run around now. Do you have any questions?"

Sonia smiled in thanks and said, "No, I understand. But I want to give you this, for your tea." Sonia handed Natalia Borisovna a small white plastic bag with a store-bought waffle cake inside. Natalia Borisovna at first resisted the gesture, objecting graciously, "No, what for? This isn't necessary." Sonia insisted, pushing the bag into Natalia Borisovna's hands, "Yes, yes, please, take it."

After Sonia left, Natalia Borisovna and I walked back to her office, and she told me about Sonia's medical history. Five years earlier, Sonia had given birth, but there had been a series of last-minute complications, including a breech delivery that was unexpected. The umbilical cord was twisted around the baby's neck, and it died a few minutes after being born. In the years since, Sonia had conceived twice more; the first time she had an abortion, and the second time she had a miscarriage at twelve weeks. The attending physician suspected the beginnings of a cancerous growth and sent Sonia to an oncologist for ongoing observation. Natalia Borisovna noted the serious character of Sonia's physical condition, and emphasized the need for her to rest and take the prescribed vitamins. Her sense of urgency, moreover, was heightened by the fact that Sonia was already thirty years old and did not yet have a child.

Natalia Borisovna had not been involved in Sonia's first birth or any of her reproductive health care since, so I wondered how Sonia had decided to come for a consultation with her now. Natalia Borisovna explained that she and Sonia shared a mutual acquaintance, a dentist who had been a classmate of Natalia Borisovna's and with whom she maintained friendly relations. This friend told Natalia Borisovna about Sonia, and the outpatient consultation was arranged. The closeness of the acquaintance link to both women, combined with Natalia Borisovna's sympathy for Sonia's case, enabled them to develop a comfortable relationship at once. Though the physician directed the conversation, she also listened attentively to her patient and met her story with an engaged concern. To express her commitment and sense of responsibility for seeing Sonia's pregnancy through to a successful outcome, Natalia Borisovna spoke to Sonia in the imagery of teamwork or collective endeavor, with herself as physician acting as "captain": "we need to get you this baby." Both her use of language and her nonverbal gestures signified a nurturing, warm, concerned feeling, conveying the explicit message that she was in charge and taking care of Sonia's needs.

In the course of the next two weeks, Sonia did admit herself to the maternity home for a few days' rest and observation. At that time, Natalia Borisovna got acquainted with Sonia's husband, Mitya, who worked as a hairdresser. Mitya offered to give Natalia Borisovna a cut and style, which she gladly accepted. The acquaintance chain started by Natalia Borisovna's and Sonia's mutual dentist friend quickly grew into a relationship of its own, characterized by gift exchanges that expressed friendship as well as mutual obligation and reciprocity. The waffle cake Sonia gave Natalia Borisovna after their first meeting, handed directly and in the context of a mutually warm, friendly interaction, was perceived by both sides as a "gift." It was followed by a series of gift exchanges between Sonia, Mitya, and Natalia Borisovna, whose relationships would continue for years. The close acquaintance link enabled Sonia and Natalia Borisovna to feel they had personalized the official, bureaucratic framework of interaction that constrained most interactions between patients and providers—the so-called "conveyor"—by mobilizing the ethically superior obligations of kinship (friendship).

Sonia returned home after a week of observation on the prenatal ward, and waited for her due date to arrive. It was early May, a time when Russia celebrates the anniversary of the country's victory in World War II. That year the holiday was celebrated with special reverence, for 1995 marked the fiftieth anniversary of the Nazi defeat. Official business in St. Petersburg closed down for three days, and the streets were filled with people watching ship parades, air exhibitions, and fireworks. On May 10, in the early afternoon I came to the hospital, where I found Natalia Borisovna and Nina Petrovna in the office, finished with lunch and drinking their tea. I greeted the physicians and asked how they had been over the last few days. Natalia Borisovna produced a faint smile and began brushing her hair; when I glanced over at her closely, she told me that she had had her hair cut and styled yesterday afternoon by Mitya, who came to the hospital. I immediately asked Natalia Borisovna how Sonia was, and—had she given birth?

Natalia Borisovna spoke in her usual matter-of-fact tone, affording me few clues for assessing her mood. "Oh yes, she sure did! Last night. Everything's basically OK."

Natalia Borisovna stood up and began washing the lunch dishes. "And is the baby OK, too?" I asked eagerly.

"The baby's basically OK, he turned around over the last week and she delivered by herself [vaginally]. There are some problems. . . . His weight was a bit low, 2900 grams, and he suffered from hypoxia due to placental deficiency, so he's in the nursery now [not in Sonia's room]. But Galina Sergeevna [the head pediatrician] said that it's not life threatening and he should be OK."

I then realized that it seemed quite remarkable that Sonia had come to the maternity hospital for a consultation, met with Natalia Borisovna, was under Natalia Borisovna's care in the prenatal unit two weeks ago, and then had given birth when Natalia Borisovna was on duty in the delivery room, a shift she had only a few times a month. Tactfully, I noted the "coincidence."

"You just happened to be on duty when Sonia gave birth?"

Natalia Borisovna looked at me and smiled somewhat sheepishly, explaining: "Maybe this is bad, but we broke her water. We had a planned induction of labor. She and I agreed on doing this because I wanted to take care of this birth. It's not that I don't trust the other doctors, but I know her and I know the situation and I had to be there to do it. We planned ahead of time that on the ninth, it was my twenty-four-hour shift, we'd break the water and start the birth."

"Well," I said, "It's important that women have people with them who know them, know their situation, their background and experiences. Especially with a person like Sonia, who has gone through so much."

Natalia Borisovna returned to her matter-of-fact, confident tone I had grown accustomed to hearing. "I had to be there. I know her and understand her. Come on, let's go downstairs together and see Sonia and the baby."

When we came to Sonia's room, we saw that a pediatrician was talking to her and her roommate, who had her baby with her. Natalia Borisovna stepped into the room, said to the doctor, "Oh, you're talking to them now? We'll come back in a little bit." Natalia Borisovna then told me we could go down to the nursery and see the baby.

First we peeked into Galina Sergeevna's office, and Natalia Borisovna asked her to come and show us which baby was Sonia's. Galina Sergeevna brought us over to the baby on the far left of the row. He had fine, light hair on his head and was sleeping comfortably. I noticed that his tiny hands appeared to be very dry, and I reached out and stroked them. Natalia Borisovna explained: "Yes, you see how dry his hands and fingers are. They're like those of an old man, even though he's just been born. They'll put cream on him and it should go away. It's due to the hypoxia, the placental insufficiency that he suffered from throughout the pregnancy. He didn't get enough nutrition."

Then Natalia Borisovna turned to Galina Sergeevna and they began discussing the baby and the birth. For the first time I realized that Natalia Borisovna was rather worried, even though she hadn't given me any hint of this until now. She looked at Galina Sergeevna and asked, "How's he doing? He'll be OK, won't he? Although of course with this placental insufficiency he's not totally OK, but what do you think?" In the hopeful but sober tone of this question I felt the fine line between Natalia Borisovna's professional interest and personal cares wane. Natalia Borisovna seemed to want reassurance herself, to know that Sonia, Mitya, and she, too, would have reason to continue celebrating.

With a friendly tone, Galina Sergeevna said warmly, "Yes, he's doing fine, I think he'll be OK. I came in and told Soniachka that I knew about everything and we may even be able to go without hospitalizing him. I'll let her come to the nursery and see him at 8 P.M."

Natalia Borisovna then reached out and touched her colleague's arm. In a tone that told Galina Sergeevna that she was asking for a favor, she explained, "Listen, last night the pediatrician on duty didn't show the baby to her, she just took the baby away—and I said, 'Look, come on, just hold up the baby, let her see him and know he's alive, that everything's OK, he's doing fine. She needs to know that and see it for herself.' That pediatrician is old and didn't think about anything; she doesn't understand much."

Galina Sergeevna listened and again reassured her colleague. "Oh no, don't worry about this. I went into Sonia's room a little while ago and said, 'My dear, everything is going well, we're taking good care of him.' She was surprised that I came to her like this, but I tried to reassure her. I think he'll be fine without being hospitalized, I mean, of course with the placental insufficiency, the brain may suffer some, it's likely that there's something there. But no, I think he's just fine."

I thanked Galina Sergeevna for letting me come in and see the baby, and Natalia Borisovna did the same, addressing her with the affectionate diminutive used between close friends and family: "Thanks, Galochka. We had wanted to go in to her, but your pediatrician was in there now, so we came by to see the baby. The doctors always tell the mothers how to care for the infants, don't they?"

"Yes, we go around after the birth and talk to them, usually in the morning. Come back any time."

Turning to leave, Natalia Borisovna said, "We'll go see if she's done in there now."

As we came back to Sonia's room, we met the pediatrician on the way out. Natalia Borisovna stopped her and asked, "Are you done in there with them?"

This pediatrician maintained a professional tone with Natalia Borisovna, and then, referring to Sonia, asked a question that showed she was not a part of the other staff's intimate circle: "Yeah, I'm done, but what's the story with that one without the baby?"

Natalia Borisovna took the opportunity to emphasize the need to treat Sonia well, to show her kindness and understanding: "Be nice to her; she lost the first one. It died after being born. Now we just have to keep her reassured that this one's alive and OK."

The pediatrician nodded with understanding, and said softly, "Yes, of course. I'm always nice to them. I'm gentle."

Several weeks later, I visited Sonia and Mitya in their home, and we discussed the problems characterizing the public health system. Sonia reiterated the appreciation and gratitude she felt to Natalia Borisovna for the care she received. I mentioned that the interactions I witnessed between her and Natalia Borisovna were uniquely warm and loving, but that most encounters between doctors and patients seemed to be riddled with conflict.

Sonia nodded her head in agreement, and explained: "Our doctors work very hard, and get practically no money in return. They're overworked, and then, as women, they go home and have to feed their families, take care of a thousand problems. Often they don't have the energy or patience to treat people the way they deserve. With acquaintances, it's better."

Sonia recognized that the constraining structure of the public health system burdened physicians' professional experiences and personal lives and largely shaped their clinic interactions with patients. Despite her own positive experiences, she was aware of the great stress and frustration that both doctors and patients experienced on a daily basis. By explaining physicians' harsh manner as an outcome of larger economic and domestic processes, her comments constructed doctors as simultaneously representatives of "our system" and victims of it. Moreover, her statement that "they're overworked, and then, as women, they go home and feed their families" revealed that she saw physicians both in their expert role as representatives of "our system" and as women, like herself, who were subject to the daily constraints of state power (as well as a system of gender difference that pervaded male-female relations). Her understanding echoed that of Elena and Olga, who insisted that rudeness and lack of personal concern were not issues of individual doctors' personalities, but reflect broader forces of "our system."

"INTERESTED" MEDICAL CARE AND PERSONAL OBLIGATIONS

As I learned in the course of time, the emotional warmth and concern that pervaded Natalia Borisovna and Sonia's interactions affected the physician as well as the patient. Natalia Borisovna carefully planned her course of action surrounding Sonia's medical care by assuming responsibility for her delivery and working at every turn to ensure that her colleagues treated Sonia well. She had not taken on Sonia's case out of self-interest or with any expectation of gaining a profitable return for her work. She threw herself into Sonia's care with wholehearted commitment out of a sense of personal obligation, initially to her dentist friend and then to Sonia herself. And she was proud of her contribution to Sonia's successful birth. The personal relationship that developed between this physician and patient thus accomplished more than transforming Sonia's experiences of a health care institution from one dominated by the constraints of "our system" to a realm of care and healing. It also provided Natalia Borisovna with the emotional fulfillment of transcending the constraining framework of "our system." She felt the professional pride of experiencing herself as a healer.

Acquaintance networks drew on the ideal concept of "*svoi chelovek*" [one of us], to designate someone with whom one shares an understanding about life and who can be relied on for personal, daily support. These relations, built on the foundation of unswerving mutual trust, stood in opposition to relations constrained by the framework of the bureaucratic machinery, with its anonymity and mass categorization of people as one of "them." Clearly, personal relations did not provide a universally accessible alternative to "our system." They were, by definition, practices of exclusion and privilege. Educational level and geographical background, nationality or ethnic identity, and other social resources provide some with a larger pool of acquaintances than others (Brown and Rusinova 1996).

Moreover, the capacity of personalizing acquaintance networks to deliver privileged care and concern, their effectiveness as strategies for obtaining one's needs, was somewhat arbitrary. My friend Karina described the following types of informal relations for accessing special care and the kinds of outcomes they tended to produce:

First, of course, is *svoi liudi* [my own people]; that's not *blat* at all but my daughter, my close friend. They will be treated as one's own relative. Then you have *blatnye doktorov*—acquaintances of acquaintances of the doctor. Midwives and other personnel won't feel any obligation to treat them specially. Then you have *blatnye administratsii*—acquaintances of the hospital administrators. They will be given a degree of special treatment, everything will be done officiously and painstakingly, but there will be no warm, caring feelings. Then you have *blatnye* for the maternity hospital itself—people who must be cared for well because they have the power to close the hospital down.

For example, Moscow established new criteria for fire safety that the maternity hospital would have to comply with. So the fire department's inspector comes to look over our hospital to check to see if we meet the requirements. Well, he tells us,

"The building isn't at all set up properly, the driveway isn't big enough for the fire trucks to get into, the escape ladders aren't properly constructed, in short—you don't meet the fire code and we have to close you down." Tamara Nikolaevna, our head midwife [a high administrative position] knows very well how to talk with bureaucrats. So she says to him, "Well, maybe there's something we can do about this?" And it turns out that this fireman has a relative who was about to give birth, and he wanted her to be taken care of by our maternity hospital. This became the highest category of *blat,* necessary for the hospital itself.

So the woman came and not only did she give birth here, but we brought her meals on a tray to her room, the chief doctor was in the delivery room with her, we did everything possible we could for her. And she was a total bitch. Her husband didn't show up sober once [*rada v zemliu*].

"Did this make everyone feel humiliated?" I asked.

"No, actually it was a unifying moment. We weren't just a few frustrated people who had to take care of her, but all of us, we unified, we all felt totally committed to managing this, so that our maternity hospital would not be closed down. 'We're doing to stay open, we'll beat this,' was the general feeling. And it made us realize that Nelly Ivanovna [the chief doctor] isn't just a bad person, she is also a victim of the system—she gets pressured and has problems from on top that trickle down to us all. It's all because of the rigid vertical hierarchy."

"Did this woman give anyone gifts of thanks afterward?"

"Nobody would ever take anything! No way. Everything's already been paid for. The fireman signed the paper and looked the other way about our building problems, so it was our turn to make sure we fulfilled our obligation. Nobody was particularly warm to her, but we waited on her. Everyone in the hospital knew. It was enough to hear, 'That gal belongs to our fireman' [*eta tetka ot nashego pozharnika*], and everyone immediately understood what was at stake."

The degree to which kindness and care would be expressed was thus influenced by the personal chemistry that emerged between persons linked by a third party (or by several intermediaries), as well as structural issues related to hospital staff relations and the channel through which a *blatnaia* gained her special privileges. Below, I explore the difficulties of attaining "good care" even through acquaintance chain networks and the fragile character of these maneuvers. The mobilization of acquaintance networks seemed the most practical strategy for removing yourself from the bonds of bureaucratized socialism, and in Sonia's case, it felt eminently moral, as well. Yet this personalizing tactic required that all involved parties systematically misrecognize the way their relationship reproduced the exclusionary character of "our system," and often failed to transcend its constraints as well.

THE CASE OF THE GREEN BAGS:
LIUDMILA AND THE REGIME OF EQUIVALENCE

An acquaintance link by itself did not guarantee a patient competent attention and kind care, but merely opened the door, so to speak, for a patient to cultivate the doctor's sense of personal obligation. Women often were handicapped by the fact that they did not know what kind of informal compensation an acquaintance doctor expected. The nature of their own relation to the acquaintance link sometimes helped, because an acquaintance might give direct instructions on appropriate compensation; but acquaintances were not always right. For a doctor longing for respect and trust, the appropriate kind of offerings—those based in sincerity— could not be manufactured.

Upon meeting Liudmila one afternoon for a prenatal consultation, Natalia Borisovna mumbled hello and in an official voice that conveyed no prior acquaintanceship whatsoever, said, "Yes, What can I do for you?"

Liudmila handed Natalia Borisovna her the medical chart and explained in a matter of fact tone, "You told me you wanted to see me at this time, so I've come back."

Natalia Borisovna manually measured the fetus and asked how Liudmila was feeling, if she had any discomfort. Liudmila was in her thirty-ninth week of pregnancy, and the conversation focused on the process of admission to the maternity hospital. Liudmila asked what she should bring with her, and what day to come.[3]

Natalia Borisovna put the fetoscope to Liudmila's uterus and listened to the fetal heartbeat, then measured the size of the uterus, first on the left side, then on the right, and on top, silently distinguishing where the fetus's limbs were. "I'm feeling here the size, he's pretty big, I'd say 3500, 3700 [grams], it's not small; definitely ready to be born [*vpolne rodivshiisia*]."

They agreed that Liudmila would come the following Monday, and Natalia Borisovna said with restrained affection, "OK, my dear [*moia khoroshaia*], get dressed."

Natalia Borisovna jotted down her notes regarding Liudmila's condition, and we all started walking out the door to the lobby.

Liudmila was clearly worried about the birth and anxious to ensure that she would have competent, attentive care. "My doctor at the prenatal clinic's not very qualified." She paused, but Natalia Borisovna did not respond. Liudmila then asked, "Are you always in the unit?"

"Yes, I'm the head of the prenatal unit; I'm here daily during the week except Saturday and Sunday, unless I come in briefly to do rounds. I also work two twenty-four-hour shifts in the delivery room per month."

Natalia Borisovna did not promise to come to the delivery, or to undertake any interventions to ensure that Liudmila would, in fact, go into labor during her shift. We reached the lobby where Liudmila's husband was waiting. As she approached, he silently handed her two green plastic bags; grasping them and turning around, Liudmila quickly extended them to Natalia Borisovna, mumbled a barely audible "thank you," and said goodbye. Natalia Borisovna took the bags without responding, turned around, and led me back upstairs. I noticed a strained, awkward expression on Liudmila's face as she handed Natalia Borisovna these bags, and I was confused as to what had just happened. "She passed you these bags in such a strange way, with such little ceremony that it was barely noticeable," I said, questioningly.

Natalia Borisovna didn't look in the bags. As we walked down the hall of the first floor, she didn't say anything at all, but only mumbled, "I'll explain it to you." As we walked up the stairs, Natalia Borisovna explained this encounter to me: "You see, I didn't want to reach out to her. I got a call from the former head of this unit who I know well, and she told me that her acquaintance would be coming by. She came for a consultation awhile ago and I examined her. She asked me, "How much do we need to pay you? We're financially well-off and just tell us how much it'll cost. We can afford anything.'"

"She thought she'd pay you personally?" I asked.

Natalia Borisovna continued with a tone of disdain:

> Me personally, the maternity hospital's administration, it made absolutely no difference to her. She just wanted to pay us money so that we'd guarantee that everything went all right. So I explained to her that we're a maternity hospital for poor women, we have no paid services, nothing is done for money, and you don't have to give me anything. I don't need anything. Well, I figured that they'd never come back, I thought I'd never see them again. And here, I guess despite it all she's decided to give birth here.

Natalia Borisovna and I walked into her office, where Nina Petrovna was sitting sewing the strap together on a worn-out sandal. From one of the bags Natalia Borisovna pulled out a hefty green box of chocolates, wrapped in plastic, with a Renoir print on the front. Judging from the packaging, this was an expensive imported box of chocolates. There was also a white plastic bottle of liqueur with a palm tree on the label and a gold elastic band around the neck with another colorful label hanging down the front and the words "Whiskey Cocktail" printed on it in English.

Natalia Borisovna frowned as she took out the items. "Here you go, another bribe [*vziatka*]. I hate getting these things. You know, they think, 'Oh, we'll give them a damn box of chocolates and that'll guarantee everything.'"

Nina Petrovna looked up from sewing and asked, "Oh, is this before or after [the patient gave birth]?"

With a look of disgust and frustration, Natalia Borisovna said only "Before."

Nina Petrovna continued sewing her sandal strap and empathized with her colleague: "Oh I can't stand that either, it's terrible. No, no, I hate that." Turning to me, she explained, "You know, they always do this, and it puts us in a very difficult position. I'm superstitious, and I hate taking things beforehand."

I sat there listening, looking at the two of them in wonder at the fact that they were complaining about it, but Natalia Borisovna had nonetheless accepted the bags.

Natalia Borisovna continued the explanation: "You know why it's a problem—[they'll say to us] 'Well I gave you [something], so you owe me—[*raz ia tebe dal, ty mne dolzhen*].'"

"Well, how would you feel if they didn't give you anything? Nothing at all?" I asked.

Natalia Borisovna hastened to respond, "It's all the same to us. I don't care. I don't need anything."

Nina Petrovna, however, was more candid about the complexity of her feelings. While not in favor of turning health care into a commodity, given the widespread poverty, she did want to feel appreciated and respected:

> You know what kills me? When afterward, they don't say, "Thank you," they just leave. No "thank you," no "goodbye," nothing. I've already gotten used to it, I don't let it bother me anymore. But you know, they could—OK, I know that not everyone can afford roses. I understand that. Three roses for some people is a really significant amount. But one rose, just one single rose, just a "thank you"—is that too much to ask?

Natalia Borisovna then handed the box of chocolates and the bottle to Nina Petrovna, who hid it away in the top of the closet, saying for my benefit, "We won't touch this now. It's better not to take anything or do anything until after everything works out. Then you can celebrate, all we want [*radi boga*]."

Liudmila's case exemplified the typical miscommunication between patients and providers. Liudmila saw her strategy as attempting to receive good treatment within the corrupt framework of the state bureaucratic system. Despite the fact that she and Natalia Borisovna shared an acquaintance who arranged an initial consultation, Liudmila still expected that she would need to "pay," reflecting the assumptions of what Ledeneva (1998: 147) calls "the regime of equivalence." Although at the first meeting Natalia Borisovna insisted that no payments were necessary, Liudmila interpreted this response as a type of posturing. At the second meeting, therefore, she came prepared "to pay," as if an unstated agreement had been established between them in the past that would govern all future interactions. Natalia Borisovna, however, resented the assumption that her medical expertise and care needed to be "bought." She felt insulted at what she perceived was an affront to her integrity as a physician, and lost any desire to establish a close personal relationship with Liudmila. "I didn't want to reach out to her," she told me. Nonetheless, by accepting the bags that Liudmila held out for her at the end of the second consultation, the physician unwittingly appeared to confirm that she had, indeed, expected such "payment."

Unraveling the distinctions between gifts of thanks and bribes required attention to the nuances of interpersonal behaviors and practices. Chocolate, liquor, and flowers were not only typical gifts of thanks in Russia, but also frequently the assumed "requirements" or "payments" for services rendered or speeded up—in short, for the special access and privileges known as *blat* (Ledeneva 1998). Consequently, subtle distinctions in the way the objects were presented became signifiers for the kind of exchange being conducted. In the maternity hospital, words of thanks or emotional warmth conveyed through a smile and gentle insistence helped frame the exchange as a "gift" of appreciation, as when Sonia gave Natalia Borisovna the waffle cake. By contrast, Liudmila's serious face, awkward glance, and uncomfortable mutter reflected her own interpretation of the exchange as an illegal payment.[4] They conveyed her view of the physician as a corrupt, bribe-taking representative of "our system," rather than as an expert endowed with legitimate authority, whose professional integrity generated automatic expectations of competent care. As a result, Liudmila's acquaintanceship appeared as a utilitarian strategy, intended to facilitate her ability to "buy" the physician, rather than to incorporate her into a moral bond of friendship and mutual obligation. And a bribe did not convey the patient's respect and gratitude, it did not transform the provider into a trusted authority, and it was not able to heal the wounds of mutual distrust.

As Sonia's story shows, Natalia Borisovna became motivated by personal concerns not merely when a patient had an acquaintance link, but when a patient sent by a close acquaintance also granted the physician authority and trust based on her stature as a medical expert. In the context of an interaction based on mutual obligations and friendship, the patient no longer viewed the physician primarily as an agent of state power; instead, she was seen through the lens of a charismatic ideology that attributed her healing power to individual knowledge and personal skill. When the bureaucratic framework of "our system" could be transcended by the

more ethical framework of a personal relationship marked by gifts of gratitude, the patient was more likely to approach the physician's dominance as
legitimate and necessary for healing, and not as the capricious, dangerous
power of an anonymous bureaucrat, a worker on the health care "conveyor." Physicians did hope that their efforts and services would be recognized and applauded; but they wanted most of all to feel that they were
respected for their skills as honest professionals and not cynically "paid
off" by patients desperate to negotiate the corrupt demands of the state
bureaucratic system. Nina Petrovna alluded to her desire for this symbolic
recognition from all patients when she rhetorically asked, "But one rose,
just one single rose, just a "thank you"—is that too much to ask?" The
irony, of course, is that the privileges extended to those with bonds of
svoi—the focused care and concern that created the trust essential to charismatic authority—reproduced the foundations of exclusion central to
"our system." The most mutually rewarding, successful acquaintance relations were founded on a profound misrecognition: the notion that the ties
that bind providers and patients could potentially be disconnected from
"our system."

YULIA'S ACQUAINTANCE RELATION: A PRIVILEGE WITH REPERCUSSIONS

Even when attended by an acquaintance physician personally concerned for their treatment, patients remained vulnerable to other hospital
staff's indifference toward this privilege, or even their resentment of it. In
Sonia's case, as we saw, Natalia Borisovna explicitly urged her colleagues to
help ensure that Sonia would be treated gently and with reassurance to
combat this possibility. She did so not by saying, "That patient's 'mine,'"
but by informing them of Sonia's tragic history and inspiring their personal sympathy. Most *blat* relations in and of themselves could not have
such powerful effects.

I first met Yulia, a twenty-three-year-old accountant, in the gynecological ward of No. 5. She had been admitted for rest and observation in
her twenty-ninth week of pregnancy, due to suspected problems with her
kidneys. Friendly and eager to talk, Yulia told me that she and her husband lived with her parents and three younger brothers in a four-room
apartment in the southernmost region of the city. At that time, Yulia
seemed to be in good spirits, even laughing about her diagnosis of kidney
problems and the apparent tensions in doctor-patient communication.
Referring to herself and her two roommates, she said jovially, "We're all
here because there are problems, they've forced us to come here (laughing); they told us all kinds of nonsense [*dogadki*] and we got scared. For

example, they told me I have problems with my kidneys. I didn't feel anything. I didn't even know where my kidneys are!"

When I interviewed Yulia more extensively at her home, however, she told me her frightening insecurity about her prenatal care, and described the events leading up to her admission to maternity home No. 5:

> When I started prenatal care, I wanted to go only to this particular doctor who is my friend's friend. She takes her time with me, and explains things. But what happened is that when she went on vacation, I had to see another doctor. This doctor looked at me and saw that I had gained weight. I mean, I had this stomach before getting pregnant, and as my first doctor said, for my weight and body size, this is normal. But when the [other] doctor saw me, she decided I was having kidney problems and needed to be hospitalized. She said that I had gained weight, was retaining water, and this was serious and I should go in for observation. I was so upset. I came home and cried. But what could I do? You realize it's for the child. So I went. But who knows, are my kidneys working better or worse? After a few days I did lose weight and the swelling went down a bit. But you know, one doctor tells you one thing, another something else. You just don't know who to believe or who to trust. You should only go through "pull" [po blatu].

Despite her sense that the bed rest helped her lose weight and reduced the swelling, Yulia did not trust the anonymous doctor. Her comment suggested that for her, authoritative knowledge resided not in science alone, but in the moral bonds of acquaintance relations. Indeed, Yulia told of drawing on her personal acquaintance networks to attain trustworthy care for every possible medical encounter without mentioning "bribery." The doctor who was her friend's friend provided personalized care both in her clinical practices and in her general knowledge of Yulia: in her words, "She takes her time with me, explains things," and, rather than relying on a standard formula of women's weight and pregnancy, knows what is normal "for my weight and body size."

I phoned Yulia two months later to hear how her birth had gone, and she immediately invited me to come over and visit. After reminding me to "definitely dress warmly" [which I saw as a sign of mutual caregiving between friends], she suggested that we take a walk with her infant daughter for some fresh air. Yulia had given birth at maternity home No. 26, because No. 5 had been closed for prophylactic cleaning during the time she was due. When I asked how she decided to give birth there, she explained that an acquaintance knew the chief doctor of No. 26, and called her to establish Yulia's connection. Arriving at the hospital five days before her due date, Yulia was assigned to a room on the prenatal ward with only one other roommate, another woman who shared an acquaintance with the chief doctor. "She came by our room and checked on us everyday," Yulia explained. "I was sure everything would go fine."

Yet in the early morning of the fifth day, when her water broke and no contractions came for five hours, the brigade on duty decided to induce labor. Yulia was confronted by the delivery room's head doctor with the snide comment, "Oh, you're here *po blatu,* so we'd better put you in a good room." They placed her in a labor room with only one other woman, while all the others in labor, about fifteen women altogether, were in one other single room. Still, the experience was traumatic:

> I couldn't move, I had to lie with my arms spread out, and the pain was just terrible. I was alone, and I couldn't move to a comfortable position; it was horrible. When they took the IV out, I walked around and moved. This helped. Then the head of the delivery room came in and she was really mean to me. She yelled at me and put the IV back in. It was so strong. I started to yell, I couldn't help it, it hurt so badly— it's scary, and you're in pain and you're alone there. And then she came in and yelled at me, "What're you howling for [*Chto ty oresh'*]?"
>
> She was obnoxious. I answered her, "I'm in pain." She said, "Oh, this is nothing," and increased the strength of the IV. When she walked away, I switched it back down again; I didn't care. Then the hospital's chief doctor came in and examined me. She put two fingers in me to see how much the cervix had opened. It hurt so much, it was just unbearable. I yelled. But the way she treated me was so understanding, so gentle. She said, "Oh, please excuse me, I know this hurts, but I'm just trying to help you." It was such a different attitude, just hearing her kind words made me feel better. But she left, and I was left with the head of the delivery room. I had mentioned to the chief doctor that they had been yelling at me, and she asked me, "Who in particular, the blond one?" I said yes, not because I wanted to get someone in trouble, but I was just in so much pain. I was worried, scared, and worried about the baby. Then when the chief doctor left, the head of the delivery room came in and said, "Oh, so now you're complaining about me!"

Yulia's acquaintance network enabled her to get partially privileged care; the hospital's chief doctor checked on her case regularly and saw to it that her conditions were more comfortable than those offered to most patients. Yet Yulia became the target of overtly hostile resentment by the chief of the delivery room brigade, the physician who was directly in charge of her childbirth experience. This doctor spared no mercy for Yulia, expressing nothing but disdain for her status as an "acquaintance-patient."

IRINA'S STORY: THE LIMITS OF A WEAK LINK

Irina's account reveals the limited effects a distant acquaintance link could have for ameliorating certain kinds of provider-patient conflicts: it would not diminish providers' sense of entitlement to weigh in on patients' reproductive decisions; nor would it address the structural constraints that engendered physicians' sense of legal vulnerability regarding—and their resulting desire to avoid—treating complicated medical cases.

I arrived at the maternity home in midmorning one day in the fall, and went to the closet to put on my white coat and begin the day. As I buttoned up the coat, Nina Petrovna and Natalia Borisovna burst into the office engrossed in a fervent discussion. With exasperation, Nina Petrovna explained that a patient in the second trimester of pregnancy had been admitted that morning due to the imminent risk of miscarrying and wanted the physicians to save the pregnancy. Nina Petrovna was furious at the request, for Irina suffered from serious chronic asthma and a heart condition. The pregnancy, Nina Petrovna asserted, not only might end in miscarriage, but was likely to endanger Irina's life as well:

> The woman has asthma, has done tests for hematology but there are still no results; she had a serious case of kidney disease. She's in danger of hemorrhaging. She's in a state of euphoria, she had a c-section the first time she gave birth, and will have one now too. And this is with the same husband! I can understand if it's not, OK, you want to strengthen the family, but I cannot understand why you'd give birth again in this condition with the same husband.

On talking with Irina and investigating the circumstances of her pregnancy, the physicians found out two social factors that they regarded as relevant for determining the medical procedures she should receive: Irina already had one child, and this pregnancy was conceived with the same husband as the first child. My confused face conveyed to the doctors that I had lost the logic of their argument. "Why does it matter whether this is the same husband or not?" I asked. Natalia Borisovna spelled out the situation: "Look, if it's a second marriage, the husband often wants a child of his own, and then maybe it makes sense to take the risk. But this is the same husband as with her first child. What does she need this baby for?!" Nina Petrovna provided an answer to this rhetorical question by rolling her eyes and holding her hands in the air as if imitating a bird flying: "She's in a state of euphoria. She's up there in the clouds, in blissful denial of the reality of her physical condition."

Embedded in the physicians' logic was the assumption that the needs of relationships motivate women to give birth: one needs a baby to keep together a marriage.[5] In this moral economy of decision-making and risk, the physicians recognized that in certain cases it may be necessary to attempt to bear a child under dangerous circumstances. Thus, upon first meeting Irina and hearing about her health problems, Nina Petrovna expected that Irina had probably just gotten remarried and "needed" to create a "new family." But given the fact that Irina was still with her first husband, the doctors declared it a huge mistake to try to bear another child. Unlike Sonia's tragedies, which threatened to leave her childless and thus aroused Natalia Borisovna's sympathy, Irina, who had one child already, was considered to be acting utterly unreasonable.

I went to Irina's room to find out her perspective on the pregnancy, her needs, and the health care she was receiving. Contrary to the doctors' perceptions, Irina was quite aware that her condition posed a danger to her own health. She had planned her pregnancy, taking out the IUD she had had inserted after her first child was born four years earlier. Upon conceiving, she immediately quit her job and was being assisted full time with the housework by her mother, who retired early in order to help her daughter. Meanwhile, Irina's husband found a second job to augment the family's income, given the loss of the two women's salaries. Moreover, the family recently had moved out of one room in a communal apartment into a two-room apartment of their own. Enumerating these details to me, Irina asserted that her family was more than able to raise a second child.

Five months later, I visited Irina at her home, a sixth-floor apartment at the top of a long, narrow staircase in a pre-revolutionary building in the heart of St. Petersburg. By this time, her infant daughter was two months old, and Irina herself had recovered from the c-section delivery, performed at another hospital. We spoke at length about her experiences with maternity hospital physicians and prenatal clinics where she had been treated. We began by discussing her experiences at maternity hospital No. 5:

> Through an acquaintance I found Nina Petrovna, and I went there when I had a threat of a miscarriage. Well, they took my temperature and realized I had a fever, so she sent me back to the prenatal clinic the next day.[6] I had to go to the primary care physician to find out if everything was OK. She said it was, that I was fine, I didn't have the flu, so I should return to the maternity hospital. But then I came back that evening, and when Nina Petrovna examined me the next day, she forgot that I had been sent there through her acquaintance, and she acted rudely toward me. I wasn't comfortable saying in front of everyone, "Don't you know, my husband gave you a present. I'm the one who knows so-and-so." So I didn't say anything. I told my husband that night, and he called our mutual acquaintance, who called Nina Petrovna. And the next day she was totally different to me.

"When you say she was rude to you, what do you mean?" I asked.

> She spoke to me using *ty* [the familiar form] and not *vy* [the formal form], and said, "Have you gone out of your mind?" Since I don't work, I am eligible for welfare services, and that's recorded on my medical history. It's written that I'm unemployed. So she said to me, "Who's supporting you to bear this child? We can give you a miscarriage if you want." So I said, "No, I came here in order to save this pregnancy." And then she said to me, "What, is your husband running around? [*Chto—muzh u tebia guliaet?*] Are you trying to hold together your marriage?"

I took that comment as a joke, but then I saw that they were serious. They said to me, "You're not being serious." My husband came later and talked to her, and then she started acting differently, once she realized who I was. But with my first asthma attack, they got rid of me.

As a native of Leningrad/St. Petersburg, Irina had an extensive network of acquaintances throughout the city. Nonetheless, she had no close links to obstetricians. Consequently, despite her efforts, Irina managed only to create a "distant" acquaintance link, one subject to being "forgotten," or even ignored in the face of a medical complication such as her asthma attack. Thus she had multiple interactions with the physicians that were characterized by insult and overwhelming alienation, as they urged her to terminate a pregnancy she desperately wanted to save.

Acquaintance chains played a role in every encounter Irina had ever had with reproductive health care. "In general, you must pay for everything in our country, either officially or unofficially."

"Can you explain what exactly happens when you 'pay unofficially'? How does it all get arranged?" I asked.

Well, what's most important is that everyone pretends that nothing is going on. You know, it's never direct and out in the open, no way. With my first child, we found the doctor like this: my husband has a friend whose wife works at the city sanitary control center. And there, there is someone who inspects maternity hospitals, and she has a friend who works in the maternity hospital where I eventually gave birth. We gave her [the inspector] a bribe [*vziatka*] so she'd talk to the doctor and convince her to do the c-section on me. You see, the person we gave the bribe to wasn't the actual doctor, but the acquaintance of the acquaintance who would go and talk the doctor into it. And it's as if nobody knows it's happening. We all pretend that it's not going on.

"What did you give this woman?" I asked.

"Flowers. Look, Nina Petrovna also got a bribe. But money isn't ever given directly to the person; it always goes through the channels of acquaintances."

In Irina's words, realizing one's needs in the public health system required "paying," and the strategy of giving flowers was called a "bribe." But Irina's characterization of the public health system contains a series of inconsistencies with the actual experiences she described having had. On the one hand, she asserted that one needs an acquaintance "to get good care," meaning both competent medicine and kind treatment. On the other hand, even when Irina found Nina Petrovna through an acquaintance, she did not assume immediate trust. Rather, in her own estimation, it was necessary surreptitiously ("as if nobody knows it's happening") to make sure the physician received flowers. Her presumption that a bribe is almost always necessary exposes Irina's almost complete lack of hope for forming mutual trust and satisfying connections with caregivers, even those found through acquaintances. This estrangement, grounded in her utter lack of faith in "our system," became the subtext of several horror stories she told me about her experiences in obtaining abortions and being treated for a post-abortion infection: "To be saved in this country, you have to do it all yourself," she stated with a quiet bitterness.

For those privileged with large networks of friends, acquaintance links offered a venue for trying to overcome the anonymity of the health care system, with its perceived indifference and poor quality care. In the best of cases, it led to improved care and a sense that biomedical power was legitimate. Yet the strategy of mobilizing acquaintance links exemplified the vulnerabilities integral to personalizing mechanisms for dealing with "our system." Inasmuch as acquaintances usually could not overcome these structural factors, they often delivered less than the patient hoped.

VALIA'S STORY: AN OBLIGATION TO PROTECT ONE'S ACQUAINTANCE-DOCTOR

My friend Valia was similarly disappointed by the care received through an acquaintance doctor, but the bitterness stung even more harshly, as this "acquaintance" was a close friend. I first met Valia and her husband in 1994, when they were setting up what soon became a very successful business in the import sector. We remained in close contact for years as I came and went to Russia, and they traveled to visit my family in the U.S. In 1999, Valia gave birth to a baby boy in one of the city's prestigious research institutes, where her friend Katya worked. Valia had actually been undergoing gynecological treatment there for some time due to suspected infertility, and Katya had arranged all her care with her most senior, respected colleagues. When in 2000 I planned to return to St. Petersburg to conduct follow-up research on paid maternity care, they invited my family and me to live with them. One rainy afternoon as we drove around the city doing errands, Valia told me of her lingering doubts and resentment about her birth process: "There's no responsibility, they're not accountable. I never heard of a doctor going to jail because they did something wrong. And they make a lot of mistakes, all the time. I still don't know if my c-section was necessary. They said the heartbeat dropped dangerously low."

"Were they listening with the wooden fetoscope?"

No, with an electronic fetal monitor. We saw the heart rate dipped. I had so much fluid, there was a lot of room for him to turn around, and he turned a few good times and got the cord around his neck twice. So they said the c-section was necessary. But it was just "quick-quick, sign here," and they thrust the papers in my face. Then one doctor, I didn't even know who he was—but I guess I could find out through Katya—anyway, he alone made the decision. Within a few seconds they put the mask on my face and I was out.

"Where was Yuri [her husband]?" I asked.

He wasn't allowed in; he waited outside the operating room door. And for two days they didn't bring the baby to me. I was in recovery, I was groggy, but still they could've told me how he was, some information about him. I lay there crying and crying, and nobody came to me, nobody showed him to me. . . . Some nurse finally brought him to me on the third day; I cried all the time, I didn't want to have a c-section. Then when I saw him I got upset because they had put an IV in his head. They said he needed it because of the trauma during the birth. Later, I asked Katya why they sewed me up so poorly. It's a vertical cut and it's very unattractive. She said it had to be vertical because it happened so quickly.

"Did Katya understand your concerns?"
"She got insulted and said, 'Look, all scars are that way. They did the best they could.' So I didn't push it further. I saw she got upset. But I feel really bad about the whole thing. Was the c-section really necessary? Will I always have to have a c-section in the future? How many times can a woman give birth by c-section—there's a limit, isn't there? It's so depressing."
"Have you considered going back and asking to see the medical records, the chart, and trying to piece together what happened, figure out if it really was necessary, maybe talk with the doctor?" I asked her. "You said Katya would be able to tell you who it was."

Well, on the one hand, I'd like to know; it would put my mind at rest. But it's complicated because Katya is my friend and it would make it difficult for her—her colleagues would ask, "Who's this troublemaker coming back and asking all these questions, stirring up problems?" I don't want to cause her problems because she really helped me and cares about me. But overall, the thing is that the doctors have power over you, and that's it. They do what they want, they don't ask you, they don't listen. They are the experts and they'll tell you what you need. And this institute is supposed to be the best. Imagine.

Valia's anger about her treatment during the birth and postpartum periods was compounded by the fact that she did not trust the medical decisions that were made. Despite the fact that she accessed this institute through a close friend who she knew cared deeply about her, this trust did not extend to the rest of the staff, including the primary doctor who took charge of her delivery and determined that a c-section was necessary. Her account of the way the decision was made—"they thrust the papers in my face . . . within a few seconds they put the mask on my face and I was out"—conveyed her feelings of remaining unconvinced about the need for, and even being coerced into, the operation. She considered the jagged scar on her stomach further evidence of the doctors' carelessness. Finally, she felt closed off from accessing additional information about what occurred during the birth: if her contact with Katya facilitated her access to this prestigious institution, it also proved an ethical obstacle to persevering in demanding provider accountability—"I don't want to cause her problems," Valia asserted. Unfortunately, Katya herself refused to take Valia's feelings seriously. She justified her colleagues' work, telling Valia that "all scars are that way," leaving Valia feeling both betrayed and guilty for criticizing her friend. For Valia knew that all scars were *not* this way. She also learned a painful, costly lesson: that friendship relations do not guarantee quality medical care, and do not necessarily override the arrogance of medical experts poised to defend their profession. Nor do they give patients systemic kinds of rights, including, at the very least, the ability to lodge complaints, have access to their charts, and file claims of negligence.

Attempts to personalize the bureaucratic framework of health care in order to receive competent medical assistance and caring attention from physicians resulted in a range of outcomes for women. In some cases, women such as Sonia, who accessed a provider on the basis of an acquaintance relation and through what Ledeneva has called "the regime of affection," experienced satisfying health care and emotionally rewarding interactions with their provider. They achieved this relationship because, first, they effectively mobilized a doctor's sense of personal obligation to treat them as a friend or relative; and second, they returned the "gift" of care with gifts of gratitude, authority, and trust— the most important and elusive forms of recognition that doctors yearned for from patients.

In most cases, however, women who aimed to personalize their health care services found that their strategy yielded mixed results at best. Yulia's acquaintance relationship with one hospital's chief doctor provided access to a certain degree of increased comfort such as a nicer room, but did not guarantee kind treatment by other hospital staff. On balance, her partial privilege carried a great cost, for it led to her sadistic treatment by another doctor who was resentful that Yulia used *blat* to obtain improved care. When women's ties to a physician involved only distant links to the doctor, it became evident that an acquaintance tie alone did not necessarily mobilize the physician's sympathy. This occurred in the cases of Liudmila and Irina, who both used an acquaintance link to try to bribe the physician for better treatment. In Liudmila's case, the bribe had the reverse effect than was intended, generating the physician's resentment and hostility, rather than a personal sense of obligation to offer better treatment. In Irina's case, the acquaintance relation was not powerful enough to be remembered, let alone inspire the doctor's sympathy, in the unfortunate situation when the patient's determination to make her own decisions about giving birth clashed with the doctor's opinions of her risks and needs.

Finally, for Valia, having a close personal friend seemed helpful in facilitating her access to an elite institution, but actually did little to empower her as a participant in her birth experience. The acquaintance-doctor offered no additional information about why a c-section was performed, and did not even acknowledge that the procedure had been done carelessly. Instead of a privilege, the presence of a close friend raised Valia's sense of personal obligation to keep her complaints private and not pursue additional answers from the hospital. Valia ended up protecting her doctor, at the expense of her own pain and lingering anger about her birth experience. As a strategy for improving reproductive health care, personalizing strategies more often then not caused a boomerang affect for women—bringing the indifference, abuse, or callousness of the bureaucratized system back to haunt them.

SIX

Privatizing Medicalization

In the fall of 1999, Yulia gave birth for a second time. I called her when I arrived in St. Petersburg in the summer of 2000, and she enthusiastically invited me over for a visit. Her elder daughter was by then almost six years old, the baby was nine months, and we spent the afternoon eagerly catching up on our lives and the changes that had occurred over the last several years. The similarities and differences between her first birth and her second were fascinating:

> I was so worried about where to go. I decided to call the chief doctor of [maternity hospital] No. 26 again. So I picked up the phone and called her at home. I said, "I don't know if you remember me, but I gave birth with you in '94 and would like to do so again." She said OK, and Max and I went there [to talk with her]. A few days before the birth I was admitted and she put me in the room "for her people" [*v palate dlia svoikh*]. Everyone, all the personnel there, know that the woman in that room belongs to the chief doctor. It was a single room, it was fine. But the most important thing was that everyone was very polite and nice, and the chief doctor came in and looked after me and the baby, and held the baby, and really worried about her. The staff, from the nurses and midwives to the doctors, everyone was very nice and helpful. For example, there are these pads you need after the birth, well, most women are in a room with five or six others, and they each get only a few pads a day. With me, they continually came in and asked me, "Can we bring you some more?" They couldn't do enough to help. Well, there was one moment when two midwives were carrying me on the stretcher, and one says to the other, "Is she a paying one?" And the other says, "Better that she's not; none of it'll ever get to us anyway." So the paid births don't help all the medical personnel; and they're doing a very difficult job for no pay.

"So how much did you pay, and how?" I asked.

"I paid $150, and I gave it to the chief doctor personally. If I had paid

at the cashier, I'd have paid in rubles, of course, but when you hand someone money personally, you give dollars. The last time I gave her a china
set."

"Do you think it's ethical to pay her money, and to pay her personally?"

"Now, I think it's a normal thing to do, and it's moral. The government doesn't allow people to make a normal salary, so this is the only way."

"How did you know what to give her? Did she tell you when you first
met?"

"She didn't tell us any sum. Max and I asked her, 'How much will it
be?' But she wouldn't name a price. She just said, 'We'll work it out later'
[*potom razberem*]. And she never told us. So we decided on our own to pay
her the same amount it costs to have a paid birth there. The only difference is that we paid her personally, not officially. But for her, it wasn't
acceptable to name a price."

* * *

Yulia's experiences offer numerous insights for understanding how
women's strategies for obtaining competent health care, and the cultural
and economic contexts of their practices, were changing by the late 1990s.
Comparing her informal negotiations with the same chief doctor in 1994
and 1999, and the different kind of interactions she encountered from the
hospital staff during her second birth, reveals some of the key aspects ac-
companying the development of paid maternity care throughout the decade. Both times, the chief doctor assigned Yulia to a privileged room
reserved for "her" patients and paid her special, attentive concern; but
during her second birth Yulia found the rest of the staff kinder and somewhat less resentful of her privileged status than they had been previously.
Another notable issue was that although by 1999 this hospital had developed an official ward for fee-for-service care, Yulia and the chief doctor
again negotiated a special, informal agreement that bypassed the hospital's
official administrative channels. Yet this time, Yulia felt that even such an
expensive gift as a china set was no longer appropriate; she expected to pay
the chief doctor personally, and in dollars, and asked her directly about the
price. Since the chief doctor neither denied the need to pay nor referred
Yulia to the cashier and the official costs, but avoided answering the question, it was clear that she expected a personal payment. But she remained
uncomfortable acknowledging this openly, and left Yulia and her husband
to figure out the appropriate payment themselves.

Investigating actual practices of paid care such as Yulia's can help shed
light on the difference between neoliberalism's imagination of market reforms in health care and the realities patients and providers confronted in

their daily lives. We have seen that Russian policymakers equated the development of patient-paid health care with the cultivation of new forms of individual responsibility among patients and providers and the improvement of health care quality. Ethnographic accounts of doctors' and patients' concerted struggles to assume personal responsibility, and rouse it in each other, allowed me to critique the assumption that neither group was motivated to care for women's health apart from economic incentives. Neoliberal reforms introduced monetary exchange as a newly legitimate tactic for accessing quality care, but largely neglected the ongoing structural impediments providers and patients faced, such as political disenfranchisement, the lack of material resources, lack of state oversight of quality, and the absence of health users' groups empowered to ensure women's rights. Moreover, stories from women like Yulia reveal that the new realm of "paid services" encompassed both official and unofficial types of arrangements, and in no way ended the use of acquaintances to secure improved care. Women explained that the state's failure to ensure adequate provider salaries partly changed the perceived ethical character of *un*official payments. In Yulia's words, it was now "normal" and "moral" to pay for care, even by subverting formal bureaucratic channels, since there was no other way doctors would earn enough to feed their families. The inability of market mechanisms alone to solve the problems of Russian providers and patients led both groups to continue deploying personal, informal strategies of care to fulfill their needs, and further led them to redefine these strategies as *moral.*

Exploring how official and unofficial fee-for-service medicine changed provider-patient relations reveals much about the cultural and economic dimensions of change after socialism. The changing cultural meanings of money reveal the shifting ways Russians provided compensation, expressed gratitude, and conveyed feelings of respect and debt as they negotiated the deployment of expert power. Paying for services holds further significance when viewed as a new cultural means of assigning and recognizing authoritative knowledge. As a symbolic articulation of legitimacy, payments at times involved women in reimagining appropriate forms of social connection. For health providers, the increasing legitimacy of monetary payments exposes changing constructions of professional identities. Integrating new practices of paying for care with familiar strategies of accessing services through acquaintances enabled both providers and patients to respond in ethically appropriate ways to the new constraints of life under market reforms, where conventional Russian notions of corruption, honesty, and right and wrong were rapidly changing. Available only to those with monetary means, such forms of morally salient change were privatized.

To speak here of "Russians" in a general sense, however, is misleading, for as the pragmatic use of money and its symbolic valences changed, they did so in different ways for providers and patients, as well as for women of different socioeconomic strata. I therefore examine three interrelated facets of the emerging fee-for-service childbirth. I begin by describing the changing institutional opportunities and constraints that shaped providers' and patients' experiences of paid services. The decentralized process of reforms, combined with a lack of state oversight, led hospitals in a scurry toward profits unregulated by protections of health users' rights. With vague standards of patient treatment, and no official criteria for selecting the providers who would work in the paid spheres, hospitals were in the advantageous position of constructing consumer demand on their own terms, rather than responding to articulated needs of informed citizens or organized workers.

Drawing on this institutional context, I explore providers' shifting notions of the kinds of exchange, recognition, and compensation they regarded as appropriate from patients. As we have seen, doctors trained during the Soviet era felt strongly about the need for providing free, universal medical assistance. As with Russians in a range of social spaces (Pesman 2000; Ries 1997), doctors treated the exchange of money as "dirty," as a sign that one's professional commitment to helping all patients was compromised. But as paid services spread throughout the medical, dental, and other service sectors, and as consumer practices became increasingly linked with signs of status and success, taking money for services gradually gained legitimacy. Earning well became not merely compatible with, but a signifier of, professional skill, a sign that one had something of value to offer. Nonetheless, very few staff had the opportunity to work in official fee-for-service care, leaving the majority of providers to accept fees unofficially (risking charges of "corruption") or remain structurally disenfranchised with neither money nor social status.

Finally, I examine patients' diverse reasons for paying for services, their official and unofficial modes of doing so, and the degree to which they found their needs fulfilled by paid care. Only 10 percent of patients had the financial means to pay for care during birth. Most of these women, however, continued to search for providers through acquaintances, explaining that merely paying money to a cashier would not guarantee better treatment and outcomes. An acquaintance-physician who also worked in a paid ward, offering both personalized concern and comfortable conditions, was considered ideal. Personal connections continued to be deployed in many cases, while informal monetary exchange—now called "payments" rather than "bribes"—gained new legitimacy as an ethical means of compensating people in a largely unethical market system.

Providers and patients alike considered monetary payments as the most promising vehicle imaginable for securing improved health care. Many spoke about payment for services as a means of overcoming system-level constraints, emphasizing the ways monetary exchanges changed people and created new kinds of subjectivities and "normal" kinds of relationships. Yet the institutional frameworks in which fee-for-service care was established both failed to resolve many systemic problems each group faced and also created new ones. Even when accessing acquaintance-physicians in paid services, many remained dissatisfied with their treatment during birth. Their stories contain frustrated, painful accounts of expert domination over decision-making, poor quality care, and feelings of total powerlessness to affect their situation. While neoliberal reforms promoted notions of individual responsibility and legitimized money, they did little to create institutional procedures or ideological recognition that state oversight and protection were necessary; as a result, reforms left open a space for unofficial payments and informal relations to persist with renewed vigor (cf. Ashwin 1999). Health care reforms reconfirmed Russian perceptions that individualized and privatized solutions, rather than institutional changes for entire collectivities, were key to fulfilling one's needs for health and well-being. Simultaneously, the disenfranchisement of both groups in political and economic terms persisted.

INSTITUTIONAL INNOVATIONS, MARKETING MANEUVERS

The maternity hospital working under WHO's Healthy Cities Project rejected the agency's ideological reforms to give women choices about birthing procedures and medical decisions. But it did incorporate WHO's technical reforms, including allowing companions during labor and instituting postpartum rooming-in with mother and baby, and it did so for every patient at no charge. In all other St. Petersburg maternity hospitals, most of WHO's technical reforms were initially defined as "additional" [*dopolnitel'nye*] services related only to patient comfort, not the quality of medical care. Throughout the 1990s, these hospitals invested their reform efforts in creating luxury wings for the estimated 10 percent of patients who were able to buy their services. Allowing companions during labor, for example, required transforming large birthing wards into individual rooms, a process that hospital administrators labeled as "costly" and as therefore necessitating patient fees. Many also constructed large private rooms for prenatal and postpartum care, with adjoining toilet and shower, television, refrigerator, lounge chair for visitors, bed for the companion, bassinet, and large changing table. This set-up presumed the presence of round-the-clock visitors and rooming-in with mother and baby, which were new and still rare procedures for Russian maternity hospitals in the mid 1990s, where the norm had always been a ward system, with babies wheeled over to mothers for scheduled feedings and a complete prohibition on visitors.

The market for childbirth services developed in a highly unregulated and uncontrolled manner, with wide variations in cost and services. During my work as a consultant for WHO in 1994, the St. Petersburg Public Health Committee took me on tours of the city's maternity hospitals, where I interviewed administrators and compared the developing path of each institution's reforms. A brief look at the various services and costs at several hospitals demonstrates the wide discrepancies between them. It is important to note, however, that most prospective patients had no access to such comparative information. Traveling across the city to investigate numerous hospitals was not feasible for the many women without a car. In interviews, women described how calling hospital information desks for information usually proved unhelpful, as most staff who answered the phones were uninformed about the paid wing's services; moreover, staff on the paid ward often refused to give out information over the phone without meeting a couple in person, a practice that suggested to many Russians that even "official" fees were subject to manipulation depending on the providers and patients in a given situation. By the end of the decade, Internet Web sites became an important source of information about birth in different maternity hospitals for those with computer literacy and access. At least one hospital had set up its own Web site to advertise its services, as we will see below, while other Web sites contained evaluations from women from throughout the city who had used one or another of the hospitals' services.

Maternity hospital No. 9 was one of the first to offer fee-for-service care, opening in 1992. Its paid ward gave women the privilege of a single, "hotel-like" room and a companion during labor, a so-called family birth. In 1994, this family birth cost 350,000 rubles (approximately $150), which provided the resources for accommodations for mother and baby and ensured the patient that a single team of personnel would treat her from the time she was admitted through the birth and postpartum periods. Out of an average of three hundred birthing women per month, approximately thirty paid for this hospital's services in 1994.

Two other hospitals (Nos. 7 and 18) told me in 1994 that they offered "hotel-style" accommodations, companions during labor, and continuity of care for a significantly lower price: 230,000 rubles ($100).[1] They regularly advertised their services in the city's newspapers and on television. Still another series of maternity hospitals were offering new services for a fee without substantially remodeling or improving their rooms. Maternity hospital No. 2 charged women a fee of 300,000 ($130) for a prenatal consultation with staff physicians and the opportunity for a companion during labor, but did not include "hotel-like" accommodations or any other privileges during their stay in the hospital. Paying women shared a room with up to four or five other mothers and their babies, divided only by a simple wooden partition. Many babies were kept in nurseries and brought to their mothers for scheduled feedings. Similarly, No. 3 offered "family births" for 180,000 rubles (just under $80), but had not remodeled to create individual postnatal rooms. These hospitals had exploited the aura surrounding the idea of "family births" and "extra services" to charge high sums of money, while actually providing fewer services than many other maternity homes, and mixing together free and paid services in the cheapest way possible. (As mentioned above, for example, the maternity hospital working within WHO's project provided a "family birth" for free, while No. 2 charged $300.)

The first years of fee-for-service care were thus characterized by a highly deregulated market that enabled hospital administrators to offer a few innovative services for whatever fees they thought they could command. While fees ranged considerably, and did not necessarily correspond with the degree of luxury or comfort provided, women had little ability to objectively compare what level of "comfort" they could buy at various hospitals. With no consumer organizations to promote fair practices, hospitals entered the competition game at a clear advantage over uninformed, disempowered buyers.

By the late 1990s, the city's Public Health Committee had shut down several maternity hospitals, citing the lower birth rate and the need to rationalize funding expenditures. Virtually all those remaining, with the exception of the hospital working with the Healthy Cities Project, instituted options for fee-for-service care as a means of raising revenue.[2] When I returned to St. Petersburg to conduct research on the development of paid maternity care in 2000, my friend Karina offered to help me update my earlier survey by calling several hospitals to inquire about their paid services. Her findings were revealing in ways I had not expected. Rather than being quoted official prices for a concrete set of "extra services," as I, a foreigner, had been six years earlier, Karina (a potential patient) received vague and ambiguous information. Maternity hospital No. 2 told her their fees approximated $300 for a "hotel-like room" with a companion present during labor and postpartum rooming-in; maternity hospital No. 9 told her that their fees began at $90 for the same services; maternity hospital No. 18 stated that their prices ranged from $200 to $500. All told her that she would need to come in for a personal consultation before any details could be confirmed. Karina interpreted this as a sign that they were seeking information on a patient's socioeconomic status in order to gauge the highest possible amount of money they could demand (a woman's and her husband's place of employment were listed on her medical chart).

The business of charging fees for patient comfort and a limited degree of choice expanded throughout the decade in both official and unofficial ways. One of the main reasons that unofficial payments continued was that providers' opportunity to charge money officially was highly restricted. Hiring in paid wards was selective (as the neoliberal model asserted it should be), but rather than based on objective criteria regarding skill, it seemed based on administrators' discretion—suggesting the exertion of favoritism. As Yulia had overheard, revenue from paid services did not augment the salaries of all members of hospital staff, but remained concentrated within the hands of a few personnel. Rather than addressing providers' collective needs for basic financial security, this system resulted in employee stratification. Many patients not only wanted comfortable conditions and a companion during labor, but sought medical care with an acquaintance; if that acquaintance did not work in an official paid ward, paying unofficially became an accepted practice. (And even if she did work in an official paid ward, many patients preferred to pay personally to ensure that their acquaintance would receive the money.)

As the decade wore on, paid wards increasingly claimed that more was available to paying clients than comfort—patients who paid money would be assured high-quality care. By 2001, maternity hospital No. 18 had posted a thirteen-page Web site to promote its "family birth ward," replete with photos of the facility and personnel.[3] This institution had one of the most highly elaborated set of services in the city, and the highest prices— "basic" paid services at No. 18 cost $700 in 2001. (The "luxury suites" were more expensive.) The Web site offers an illuminating insight into the kinds of innovations and improvements the staff themselves construed as constituting care worthy of payment. Indeed, by articulating its official offerings and fees, this Web site exposes how an emerging neoliberal model of "service" constructed consumer demand in Russian childbirth. The site greeted visitors with the following lines:

> What does your family dream of while awaiting the arrival of the baby? Well, of course, that the baby will be totally healthy, the birth will take place successfully, and, to the extent possible, painlessly. Do you want to guarantee yourself safety, the professionalism of the staff, good conditions during your stay at the maternity hospital, and the timely attention and proper attitude of the staff? Do you dream of giving your baby all the best? We offer you—from the very beginning—all the best for you and your baby![4]

While promising a "safe" birth, the basis of the "guarantee" remains notably vague. The site presents no statement of patient rights or legal backing of this "guarantee," and no comments about compensation or redress in the case of patient complaints. Rather, the site details the special medically related services available to paying clients: the cost of prenatal hospital stays in the "family" ward if medically necessary, choice of a single doctor for all stages of birth, a course on childbirth preparation and adjustment to parenthood, psychological counseling about the birth process and the father's role in it, and training in biofeedback for relaxation and pain relief. There were far fewer details about the actual medical procedures and the staff's approach to the birth process. The text stated: "Individual delivery with the husband present occurs under the new, kinder and gentler method, which minimizes trauma to the mother and newborn (we do not break the water, do not induce births, and use minimal medications), vertical positioning during birth (at your desire)."[5]

The vague, general nature of the information provided to the public about the procedures surrounding labor and delivery works to ensure that patients remain uninformed about precise medical procedures. The text consistently focuses on "service" kinds of issues, describing, for example, round-the-clock midwifery care, daytime nursing care, and daily exams by the obstetrician and neonatologist. Such specialist care was standard procedure in free wards too, but the unstated assumption was that treatment would be more attentive and competent for those who paid. Additional "medical-physical services" for the mother included postpartum exercises, a mini solarium, a cosmetologist, and a hair dresser (2001: 8). The hospital offered anesthesia during birth "at your desire," but the basic cost of $700 did not cover epidurals unless medically indicated. With this, the discussion of "medical services" ended. As the text continued, its main focus concerned comfort—now elaborated with the English term "service" [*servis; servisnye uslugi*], intended to signify a Western-style, consumer approach. The text cited comfortable conditions of the delivery rooms, its "modern equipment" for mother and child, and the paying patient's guarantee of medicines and disposable materials, from sewing materials (presumably to repair tears or episiotomies) to bed sheets (2001: 5). Implicitly contrasting its offerings with the shortages found in "free" medicine, the text enumerated all available supplies for mother and child, including full sets of bed sheets (and additional ones for the relative), diapers, and hygienic supplies. It highlighted and posted photos of the ward's comfort facilities, including "a cozy café, a lounge, video player, television, buffet, and telephone" (2001: 8). Patients' needs, it was implied, were limited to the social-psychological aspects of care, such as kind attention and pretty, comfortable surroundings. Medical decision-making would remain the

province of professionals. There was no comment that women had rights
to information about the medical procedures being undertaken. Patients
were constructed as buyers entitled to receive quality services, but not
active participants in decision-making concerning the birth process.

The one section where women were not depicted as passive recipients
of care, ironically, depicted women as largely responsible for the outcome
of birth. Encouraging women to take their birth preparation course, the
hospital then warned:

> The length and safety of the birth process, and the level of pain, are in many ways
> determined by how you are disposed [*vashem nastroem*], your proper behavior, your
> skill in self-regulation (preparation for birth). Much during the birthing period
> depends solely on the woman herself, on what she is able to mobilize herself to do as
> she thinks about her child, his safety, her ability to fulfill all the necessary tasks, and
> relate to this as difficult, responsible, and creative work. (2001: 8)

To say that women themselves bear responsibility for the length, safety,
and painfulness of labor and delivery elides the roles of both nature and
medical interventions in shaping the birth process. This move reconfirms
cultural notions that women need to "take responsibility" for their health,
without acknowledging the ways broader systems within both the health
care structure and society at large enable or impede this ability. The Web
site concluded by appearing to offer the woman support, defining her as
an "active agent" and the experts as "loyal and reliable helpers." Yet without encouraging women's participation in medical decision-making by recognizing, for example, the contested scientific status of certain medical
procedures, such as the use of episiotomies, criteria for caesarean sections,
and diagnoses and prescriptions for eclampsia, these terms seem largely
rhetorical. Women can hardly be "active agents" in a process where they
have no opportunity to weigh in on the central medical issues of their
birth experience. The "full support" promised women seems reserved for
those who comply with medical power, or in the words of the text, display
"proper behavior."

DOCTORING WITH DIGNITY, WITH MONEY

When fee-for-service care became possible in the early 1990s, many
doctors first responded with ambivalence. Accepting monetary payments
offered opportunities for better equipment and economic stability, on the
one hand, but raised a whole host of ethical concerns, on the other. In
1994–95, and even as late as 1998, physicians I interviewed from hospitals
throughout St. Petersburg felt compelled to reassert the integrity of their
professional commitments, claiming that what was available to be pur-

chased was not their competence, but medically unimportant issues such as a private room. Even while this claim changed in hospitals' promotional work, as we have just seen, the need to establish their professional integrity continued to be a key source of anxiety for physicians. Several related ethical issues emerged.

One area of tension was that working in paid services was clearly a privilege, which created new forms of stratification between medical personnel. Hospital administrators bestowed the opportunity to work on paid wards on staff of their choosing; no official criteria existed for who would get to earn higher salaries. In other words, the introduction of official forms of payment was not done in a way that repaired the sense shared by all physicians that their work was undervalued. It extended the official system's preexisting injustices to create new forms of inequalities between hospital staff.

Another ethical dilemma many physicians faced was the prevailing notion that taking money for medical services was morally wrong. These doctors equated professional dignity with an ethic of healing and caring from the heart, a perspective opposed to "doing business." In 2000, while I was visiting with a friend, Alexei, his life-long friend Leva, a committed doctor whom I had met on a few occasions before, suddenly dropped by. "How are you doing?" I asked casually, not having seen him for several years. Unaccustomed to American-style small talk, Leva plunged into the difficulties of his professional life.

"I make 582 rubles a month," he answered with a melancholic smile that conveyed the despair of living a life of absurdity. "I work nights in the hospital as a surgeon fixing broken bones, appendicitis, and doing other kinds of surgical procedures. I work eight hours a day. To make extra money, I work twenty-four-hour shifts throughout the month, and my salary usually gets up to 1,500–2000 ($53–$71.) Just to survive, I work as a postman on the days I'm not at the hospital. In three days I can make as much as in the hospital all week."

I stood there looking at Leva aghast. I asked Leva if his patients at the hospital gave him gifts of thanks. "Very rarely. Maybe in one out of twenty or thirty cases. You see, they're a special sector of society; many have come from prisons. They have all kinds of problems, HIV infection. But in maternity hospitals, I know, to get any attention paid to you at all, you must pay the doctor directly in his hand, and in dollars."

Leva said this in disgust—it was dirty, immoral, a breakdown of all appropriate, decent standards for physicians, his tone conveyed. "I try to get some private patients of my own. Sometimes they hear of me through my acquaintances. I give massages and treat all kinds of problems. But I can't name a price. I just don't, it's not my way. People have different abilities, and they pay what they can. They know how little I make."

For Leva, as for the chief doctor that Yulia described, it was wrong, even morally transgressive, to name a price for his care; whatever they pay, even nothing, he accepted. This was his vision of being a doctor, a healer. "Maybe you could do massages for rich people," I suggested, offering him a way of making more money. "I don't want to give massages to rich people," he said categorically—"I need to work with people like me, on my level. I need to feel I share a basic understanding with the people I treat. Wealthy people, they're different, they're a different type. No, I wouldn't give them massages."

I found many physicians who expressed ambivalence about taking money from patients, but by the end of the decade, most came to view it as a necessary evil. In a revealing conversation I had with the chief doctor of a women's outpatient gynecological clinic, Valentina Pavlovna explained that she had instituted fee-for-service abortions to anyone willing to pay. In the entrance to the clinic, a list of services and their prices was posted on the wall that included the offering of "paid abortions." Women with residence permits in the catchment area of the clinic were eligible for free abortions, but, Valentina Pavlovna explained, women often *wanted to pay.* When asked to explain the difference between paid and free abortions, she immediately responded: "With paid services, you get the best doctors."

My acquaintance from the Public Health Committee pressed her further. "Can you guarantee they're the best?"

"Well," Valentina Pavlovna admitted, "the women think there's a guarantee." She paused, evidently uncomfortable with the ethical challenge the discussion raised. "I can't do bad work," she concluded with a tone of insistence. "Sometimes I even do more for free than for those who pay." In these comments, the chief doctor revealed several important issues. First, she exposed the fact that an unregulated market in Russian health care has not simply led to a higher quality of care, more dedicated providers, and increased efficiency. Clinics have exploited the widespread consumer dissatisfaction with the quality of free care, combined with the lack of public information about health care reforms and the lack of state oversight, to turn a profit. Second, when Valentina Pavlovna backtracked to assert, "I can't do bad work," she also implicitly contested the neoliberal assumptions touted in Russian public health journals that doctors would be "interested" in the outcomes of their work only if well paid. For this Russian doctor and many others, at stake in the issue of whether women who paid actually obtained a superior quality of care was the question of whether their competence and professional dedication were available *only* if *bought.* While Valentina Pavlovna had based her clinic's new incarnation largely on the popular acceptance of this assumption, she was unable to confirm it as true.

By 1998, many physicians I had known since 1994 felt less ambivalent about taking payments and even doing so informally. Several factors influenced these changes. Paid services had become very widespread throughout the health care system. The colloquial expression "we pretend to work, and they pretend to pay us," which had captured so perfectly the frustrations of work life during the Soviet era, no longer seemed the inevitable arrangement. In August of 1998, the ruble crashed, and the material situation in and outside hospitals worsened considerably. As described in earlier chapters, the maternity hospital where I conducted fieldwork did not have sufficient amounts of essential medical supplies; doctors routinely had to tell women to purchase their own antibiotics and other medications and bring them to the birth. The hospital often had no hot water. Personnel, including doctors, were required to work after hours trimming the bushes and picking up garbage on the hospital grounds. Just after the ruble crashed, St. Petersburg was hit by extensive floods. Hospital personnel were called to bail water out of the maternity hospital's basement, which they did for a week straight, again with no compensation. Much of the sheet supply was ruined, and there was no money to replace it. Patients would now have to bring their own sheets in addition to medicines. The state was abdicating its role in supporting health care, and doctors came to feel that they no longer had to continue "working for free." Nor was it a really possible to do so any longer. Providers needed money for daily life needs—for their children's textbooks, higher education, and even health care. They viewed the failure of the state to provide the necessary resources for public health—to fulfill its basic obligations—as the foundation of "corruption," and a reasonable justification for bypassing the laws to accept unofficial payments.

Doctors also felt that women showed more compliance when medicines or procedures cost money. The very existence of a price seemed to signify value, as opposed to "free" care, I heard repeatedly from a range of people, from elites such as the deputy chief of the city's Public Health Committee to my close friend Karina. The chief doctor did not agree. The overwhelming majority of women were poor and could not afford to pay for care, she argued. Moreover, the establishment of distinct levels of comfort and care under the rubric of paid services was unjust, both to poor patients and to hospital staff. Women birthing on the paid ward would surely need the services of some staff from the free section, and how could compensation be fairly distributed? Envy and competition were sure to result, she claimed. Providers, however, perceived the prohibition against charging fees as deeply unfair, given that their colleagues in all other city hospitals had started doing so. Moreover, as Natalia Borisovna told me in 1998, doctors constantly encountered patients who *asked* to pay them personally. Refusing such offers increasingly seemed absurd and unfair, "because we get all types of patients. Some arrive and leave in a Mercedes, while we doctors walk home on foot."

When I met with Natalia Borisovna again in 2000, she alluded to the fact that paid services had become entirely legitimate (though I knew they were still officially prohibited by her chief doctor): "We've now matured to the point [*my uzhe sozreli do togo*] where we understand the need for paid services, and how to undertake them." She did not go into details, but another physician on staff explained to me that several doctors had established an underground, informal system offering the services of a "personal doctor" [*lichnyi vrach*] to trusted acquaintances of acquaintances. This business-type arrangement built on earlier personalizing relations of the type we saw with Sonia, but now the doctor gave the patient her beeper number, told her to call when labor began, and promised to attend the birth as the patient's own doctor. The compensation was monetary, and the price made known through the acquaintance. Still, this informal practice could be undertaken only by the more senior, respected doctors on staff, those who could garner the support of auxiliary personnel essential for realizing their promises to patients.

My friend Galia, an obstetrician-gynecologist working toward a Ph.D., underwent changes in values similar to Natalia Borisovna's. I first met Galia when she worked at one of the city's women's outpatient clinics in 1995, and we began spending time together during her work and on the weekends. That year, an American acquaintance of mine also conducting research in St. Petersburg needed the assistance of a gynecologist, and I contacted Galia, knowing that she would be kind and communicative. To express our gratitude for her help, I brought Galia a waffle cake from me and this friend a few weeks later when I had the chance to see her again. As I explained how appreciative we were and held out the bag with a warm smile, she initially reacted with horror, "No, no, you don't need to give me anything!" she cried, construing the offering as a "payment." Recalling Sonya's encounter with Natalia Borisovna, I did my best to reassure Galia that my friend merely wanted to thank her for her time and understanding, and asked her to please take the gift in that spirit. I felt quite worried about having insulted her, but when Galia looked into the bag and saw that it was, indeed, only a modest waffle cake, her face lightened up and she smiled gratefully.

Three years later, in June 1998, I lived with Galia and her young daughter in their St. Petersburg apartment for two weeks. By that time she had defended her dissertation and was now working in one of the city's prestigious medical institutes teaching and conducting clinical work. Her attitude toward money had changed dramatically: "My salary is pretty good for a doctor: I make 770 rubles a month, about $120."

"But how can you live on that?" I asked.

"Well, not just anyone will come to be treated at this institute; it's very prestigious. The people who go there are willing to pay for their treatment, so this gives us a chance to make some money."

"So you work in paid services?" I asked, somewhat confused.

"Well, some pay [through that] but from those payments, official payments, we don't earn anything. . . . [Other] people ask an acquaintance, and she'll set it up beforehand and ask if it's possible. They call ahead and find out the cost. I don't take money from someone off the street. It could be, you know, like a set-up, watching you."

"So you get paid pretty much all the time through acquaintances?"

"I'll see anyone once, for a consultation. I won't necessarily take money —if the person can't pay, they can't pay. But I won't do it twice. She can go to any clinic and get treated for free. If she wants to come here, she has to pay. I respect my skills and my time too much not to take money [*Ia uvazhaiu svoe vremia, svoiu kvalifikatsiiu*]."

This assertion represented a profound change in the cultural logic of professional integrity. If Soviet and Russian notions of monetary exchange had long been tainted as morally reprehensible—and a waffle cake was viewed as the appropriate way to express gratitude to an acquaintance-doctor—Galia had now come to consider monetary payment as the expected remuneration for her time and skills. No longer indecent, polluting, and blasphemous, money had become a key component of her professional identity and sense of integrity. Still, the fact that payments remained unofficial posed a constant threat to this legitimacy:

> Everyone takes money, everyone. But it's not official. Look, yesterday I had an interesting experience for you. A woman I've been taking care of throughout her pregnancy called me; she's thirty-seven weeks pregnant and even though mostly the pregnancy has gone fine, she was told by someone that there were suddenly all kinds of problems. So I told her to come in and I checked her out. I did an ultrasound. Things seemed to be not so bad, but I wanted to be absolutely sure. So I asked another doctor, an older colleague with a lot of experience, to take a look. Her name was Maria Ivanovna. So she examined the woman and, as I thought, said that she was OK and there was no need to be admitted. Now, this was the first time I had ever consulted with this Maria Ivanovna. When the patient came and gave me a hundred rubles, I wasn't sure what to do. I thought, well, I shouldn't give her all of it because she didn't do that much, but after all, she did examine her. But on the other hand, I didn't think it was necessary for her to know I took money from this patient. I mean, everyone takes money. And everyone knows everyone takes money. But if I came to her and gave her fifty rubles, then she'd have proof that I took the money. I didn't know what to do. So I went to another doctor, a pediatrician who I know, and I asked her what to do. She said, "Don't do anything." Because if I gave Maria Ivanovna fifty rubles, she'd probably go spreading the word to everyone that I took money. That's something I don't need.

By 1998, the informal language of respect for expertise had been wide-ly translated into the idioms of monetary payment. If in 1995 Natalia Borisovna and Nina Petrovna expressed resentment when Liudmila assumed that a payment would be expected, and Galia responded with shock to the thought that my acquaintance and I would give her a "payment," these doctors now viewed the receipt of money for one's work as a necessary condition for not being exploited. Yet in the many cases where physicians were not authorized to accept money for services, they had felt forced to choose between two unsatisfying positions, both of which undermined their sense of respect and recognition in this new moral economy: on the one hand, they could accept money informally and acquire the feeling that their work was respected, but in doing so they would need to break the law, and would risk being exposed as "corrupt." On the other hand, they could refuse to take payments, enjoy the safety of one who follows the rules, but remain excluded from emerging sources of symbolic status and material necessity. When the legal framework itself seemed so unjust, deciding on the latter course felt nothing less than foolish.

Finally, it should be pointed out that as providers such as Natalia Borisovna and Galia faced these ethical dilemmas about participating in fee-for-service care, they were left to negotiate these emerging practices in informal, privatized ways. When policymakers aimed to stimulate worker productivity and quality by instituting economic incentives alone, they failed to address providers' political needs to define and defend their occupational interests. The neoliberal service model, in other words, left issues of collective justice for workers invisible. With no forum for negotiating collectively with policymakers and administrators about the terms of official, fee-for-service care, the state essentially invited informal strategies, "unofficial payments"—to expand. In turn, doctors justified unofficial payments ideologically through discourses demanding individual responsibility from patients. Rather than viewing patient "choice" as a universal right, Natalia Borisovna, Galia, and others argued that each person has the obligation to assume responsibility for her health by seeking out personal relations with doctors she trusts, and privately compensating them.

PATIENTS' STORIES

When paid services became possible, many women hoped they would be a key means of motivating doctors to provide individualized attention. Patients often spoke of money as necessary for obtaining "good service," for "motivating" doctors. Interestingly, I found a difference in the symbolic significance of money for women of different classes. Women with limited resources regarded money as a simple necessity for obtaining quality care; they spoke of paying for services in pragmatic terms alone. Affluent women connected to the business world, by contrast, insisted on the legitimacy of payment for services as an element of a new, post-Soviet worldview. They frequently reified high prices as charismatic proof of a physician's true medical competence, rather than as a reflection of her connections and privileges.[6] Thus, one woman I interviewed told me that if a provider did not name a price for her services, clearly the doctor had little of value to offer. This woman did not consider other possible reasons for not charging money—such as being prohibited to do so by one's superiors, or lacking the requisite connections to do so informally, or being committed ethically to providing free health care. Still, the majority of women interviewed who used paid childbirth services between 1992 and 2000 found themselves barely any safer than in the free wards.

Masha's story was the happy exception. I begin with her account because her sense that she had a wonderful birth experience helps illuminate the kinds of concerns and needs some women had, and the evaluative criteria they applied to judging how their experience went. Moreover, Masha emphasized that she hoped I would use her story in my book to show that there were committed professionals in Russia's maternity system, people fully dedicated to making the birth "a celebration for everyone." Masha was twenty-six years old at the time of her baby's birth and had a degree in journalism and a job with the city's main television station, but decided not to continue working after the birth. Her husband's income was comfortable, and he had high connections in the city government. In fact, Masha found a maternity hospital through acquaintances whom her husband met at work. She explained that she did not search for a paid ward per se, but a place where the care would be good. Fortunately, a chance encounter during the last months of her pregnancy directed her to the right place. Masha explained:

> Vitali [her husband] had the opportunity to meet the head of maternity care services in the St. Petersburg Public Health Committee. She could feel how worried we were, how important it was to us, that we weren't just—she saw what kind of people we were—and that's important—and she said, "I'll tell you, there are two maternity hospitals that I'd give birth in myself." These are simply people who're trying—with all that's going on in our city with public health—to work—not out of the desire for money, but out of naked enthusiasm—to build what they imagine should exist. It turned out there was an absolutely amazing chief doctor in one hospital's paid ward.

Masha met with this doctor and toured the paid ward soon after meeting this city policymaker. She was thrilled with its beautiful décor and equipment. She described the atmosphere of the ward in almost fairytale fashion:

There was a totally amazing rose-pear color to the corridor, ten rooms, two delivery rooms, and two pre-delivery rooms. With their staff, eight obstetricians and one midwife, they're all young, they do it all. They have their own laundry, they wash everything, the full set of sheets, and most important, an iron. They create this atmosphere where every morning they brought me a starched set of sheets, diapers, shirts, robes, everything you need. And who irons and washes—they do—from the director to the nurses, whoever has a free minute, everyone stands near that iron and irons the clothes and sheets.

During the tour, she met the staff, and then filled out the paperwork and paid her money. The chief gave her the phone number of the ward and her own home phone number, and told her to be sure to call when the birth began, or at any time she had questions or concerns.

When Masha's contractions began late one night two weeks before her due date, she called the ward, and they told her to catch a taxi and come right over. She entered the hospital through the general admitting room for all patients:

When I got to this admitting room where everyone goes, there was this totally horrible, ragged gal, who didn't say hello or goodbye, just—"Where's your chart, sit down, blood pressure," and my water begins to break, I feel I'm wet. I tell her, and then suddenly a totally amazing girl rushes in, with a beautiful figure, ironed and starched uniform, and says with reassurance, "Mashinka, now, now. I'm taking you, don't worry." She takes my things and the other one looks at me like, "Oh, she's paying." My girl smiles at me and takes me up the elevator to an entirely different world, and they put me in absolutely wonderful clothes—I never saw such starched night clothes. They changed me every twenty minutes, a new shirt, and new robe, because I kept getting wet.

The shift changed in the morning, and the doctor who had been with Masha throughout the night told her, "Don't worry, another girl, an obstetrician, Elena, is coming. She's very good. Don't be afraid."

And Elena comes in and I was really enchanted by her. How they pick the[se doctors], I don't know, [but] they have as much on the outside as on the inside. These people have such qualities—they're so sympathetic, young, she was a twenty-six-year-old girl. Not straight out of medical school. They can do it all. They don't avoid any tasks, all of them, from the cleaners to the classy doctors. And she immediately reached out to me, she'd just come off an all-night shift, and she delivered me. And at the end, the chief came in and said, "I'll sew you up myself."

"Why do you think it's so good there, and so bad in the general ward?"
"Because they love their work. It's because of that they were chosen to work there. It wasn't arbitrary that they chose these people to form this

team. They choose people for whom money is absolutely not necessary. Well, how do I explain it? It's not that they don't need money. They're all young girls, who want . . ."

"To dress well, go out . . . ," my research assistant, Irina, interjected.

"Yes, but their work is the most important thing to them and they don't need anything else in life. That was the impression I got, I spoke with them. . . . None of them yet had families of their own. It seemed they all had just work on their minds. They wanted their team to make the best maternity hospital. These people had a goal."

"And why do you think it was so bad in the free ward?"

"Because the people there, maybe, had professions they didn't want."

"Well, nobody forced them into it."

"It's everywhere like this. When I was admitted to the hospital for two weeks for observation, there was a cleaner who makes 160 (less than $27) a month. She was so rude to us. . . . I think if you agree to work at that job and for that amount of money, you have to work right."

"The money you paid, did it go to the cashier?"

"I know where it went. I spoke with the director. I paid about 3000 ($500). One hundred rubles (less than $17) went to the midwife. Some small amount went to the development of the ward, and all the rest to the entire maternity hospital. This ward, God willing, gets 10 percent of the total sum. They don't have anything. They don't need money, as I later found out, because the midwife only got 100 rubles out of my money for all her work with my birth."

"Were you satisfied with the birth, with the treatment?"

I felt like I was the most important person in it all, that we were working together for one thing. . . . I tried to do things so that they'd praise me. They praised me, said, "That's right, good going, you're doing great, you're holding out terrifically." Everything went according to the textbook. I didn't have any complications, and when it was all over, the director immediately came running up to me and said, "When'll you come back for the second one?" And she even began stroking me on the head, and I kissed her hand, it was all like that. I said, "Thank you so much. I'm so happy."

Upon being discharged, Masha thanked each of the staff personally and with great warmth. Her husband brought an enormous bouquet of flowers for them. "Well, you're not going to just give money, it was clear that they wouldn't take any money, they were just happy everything was OK."

"Did you give any gift to the woman from the Public Health Committee who originally referred you there?"

"No, she has a pretty high position and to distract her a second time would be inappropriate. I think Vitali called her and said, 'Many thanks, everything worked out fine.'"

Masha also told of several friends who had delivered on paid wards and had negative experiences. When asked what caused the problems, she again linked staff attitudes with the character of people working on the wards: "It turned out to be a place where they take money for the sake of money, and the people haven't changed at all [*a liudi vse prezhnie*]. The brigade who delivered one friend also worked on the free ward, and psychologically, they haven't changed. They howl at everyone on the free ward, and they do so on the paid ward. There's not this separate microclimate."

"Do you think the wonderful experience you had was affected by your going through contacts, through the Committee of Public Health?"

"Well, I think that had a little effect. Yes, of course, there was greater attention because they had the call from the Committee. But then when I was there for ten days, I talked with all the girls on the ward, and I saw that everyone had it well. Everyone had it good and there was an attentive attitude toward everyone."

Masha looked for a maternity hospital that came recommended, not necessarily one that had paid services. Her satisfaction with her birth stemmed from the caring interactions and aesthetic conditions she experienced. She had no complaints and rather few comments about the medical procedures undertaken; but she did comment repeatedly on the beauty of the ward, the plentiful supplies, and the aesthetic quality of the clothes (note her enthusiastic emphasis on the starched, ironed clothes of the staff and patients).

Masha stood out among interviewees with her refusal to connect her positive experiences with the money she paid. She insisted that staff on this ward were enthusiasts fulfilling their dream to create a superb maternity hospital. She asserted they "didn't need" money, and presumed they "wouldn't take it" had she offered additional payment as gratitude upon leaving. She expressed no doubts about the chief doctor's assertion that 90 percent of the revenue from the paid births went into the general upkeep of the hospital, and did not question the ethics of paying the midwife only 100 rubles out of the total fee of 3000. People who did not earn much obviously "didn't need money," she reasoned. Her image of the staff working as a team for idealistic goals alone implicitly rejected the possibility that any conflicts or even division of labor stratified them, as in her comment that everyone, "from the director to the nurses, whoever has a free minute" irons. If this group was chosen because of their enthusiasm and commitment, their deep human sympathy, they stood in contrast to the ragged look and rudeness of personnel in the free wards—characteristics that she similarly portrayed as reflecting their personality traits—and their apathy toward their work. In explaining the rudeness of staff in a paid ward in another hospital where her friend went, she cited their psychologically unreconstructed behavior, and labeled them as "anachronistic people" [*liudi vse prezhnie*]—as if "changing with the times" was solely a matter of individual choice, unaffected by one's larger political-economic conditions. Thus, while Masha refused to attribute her positive experience to the money she paid, her assessment of health care quality continued to rely on a logic of individual, rather than systemic, change. Personal commitment was key to improved care, no matter what sorts of external conditions prevailed.

OKSANA'S STORY

If Masha rejected the idea that money could be a motivating factor in providing high-quality care, Oksana believed it was the key to securing improved services. Hers is a story of someone who attempted to free herself from the "dependency" that personal obligations created between people. Oksana gave birth in 1994, just months after maternity hospital No. 18 opened the doors to its paid ward. Thirty-one years old, with a Ph.D. and a husband with a lucrative salary, Oksana had a precise image of what she wanted from her birth experience:

> I wanted a normal delivery room, in which no other patients were around, attentive care, and for my baby to be born in the best conditions. Plus, I wanted the baby to be put to my breast immediately, for the baby to be with me, and not to be left somewhere screaming. I didn't want them to give him any sleep-inducing, supplemental feedings so he wouldn't scream and wake up the attendant. That's what I expected.

To find an appropriate hospital, Oksana and her husband visited several of the hospitals with paid services and spoke to everyone she knew who had information about them. Negative experiences with hospital staff began at that early point. While consulting with the administrator of one paid ward, she sat at a table while the doctor looked over her chart—and then wrote new diagnoses in it: nephritis and pre-eclampsia.

"Did she examine you?"

> Not at all. We sat at the table. She looked at my chart from the prenatal clinic, which already listed me as an "old mother," and just made these things up. I knew then I would never give birth there. But then I couldn't go back to the prenatal clinic with these new diagnoses written there. So I threw my chart in the trash and told the prenatal clinic my purse had been stolen with it in there. They had to write me up a new chart, and I had to find another maternity hospital.

Oksana had a few links to acquaintances at other maternity hospitals, but decided not to go that route. "My thinking was that if I go through normal channels and I pay a normal amount of money, I should receive a normal kind of interaction. I didn't want any favors when I was able to pay. Why should I have to ask for something when I can pay and be in an absolutely independent position, not dependent on anyone?"

So Oksana visited No. 18 and was immediately impressed:

> I went there and saw young women, you know, young, well-dressed, with normal hair cuts and normal faces (laughs), not impudent [*khamskie*] women. They had a normal manner of speech, used normal language. That meant something to me. I thought, yes, they were modern, you know. I think that factor was decisive. After I decided I'd give birth there, we went back and I paid my money—it cost $200. About two weeks later, I went again and the ward's chief examined me and we agreed that if she wasn't on duty when I gave birth, we'd call her at home and she'd come in specially for me. I asked her if we could make this arrangement, and I let her know I'd pay her extra for it. . . . But it turned out she was on duty.

"So you didn't pay more than the official sum?"

"We left a bouquet of flowers and a cake, I left it for the ward. I didn't pay anything more. And I'll tell you why. I was dissatisfied with the birth."

"Why weren't you satisfied?"

"Because I was too well prepared, for one. On the other hand, I'm a perfectionist, I wanted it to be superb. . . . I showed them this big American encyclopedia and said, 'I want to deliver like that.' On a bed, not in gynecological stirrups."

"This was when you arrived to give birth?"

> Yes. I felt totally fine. I said I want to do it this way, only this way. OK? OK. So I'm walking around the halls, there was another woman in the ward who'd been induced and was yelling, and I didn't want to hear it. But the midwife came over to me at noon. She said, "Come on, your contractions began at 12 A.M., and now it's noon, so let's go." My water hadn't broken. She says, "Let's go break your water." I asked her if it was necessary, and she says, "Yes." And she breaks it and there's meconium in the fluid. So she says, "There's a pathology, the baby could choke—you need to get on the gynecological chair. (in stirrups)" I say, "Let me do it on the bed." "No, on the chair." And as soon as I got up there, my need to push ended. It was total idiocy.
>
> Why [do you think] women don't want to go to the gynecologist? Why are women afraid of the gynecologist? Because each time you sit on that "helicopter," excuse me, it's rape (laughs). Every time—sex. Yeah. They rushed because they were worried the baby was going to choke. And the baby was born and they went to dry him off on the towel and the neonatologist says to me, "Look, you see how he came out, with closed eyes," as if he was an unfortunate, tortured baby.

"And what, you were to blame for this?"

"Naturally. I remember, I said, 'Put him with the cord attached on my breast.' The neonatologist said, 'No.' They first washed him, swaddled him, and then put him on me. And they gave me an episiotomy—I was categorically against episiotomies. But they did it anyway. I remember precisely yelling, 'Why are you cutting?'"

"Did you tell them that ahead of time?"

"I told them a thousand times. But they cut me anyway. It's always like that here. The road to hell is paved with good intentions."

"So why'd they do the episiotomy?"

"They said that the last ultrasound showed the baby was going to be four kilos. He was born at 3100 grams. He'd have been able to go through entirely normally."

"How was their attitude to you overall? How did they interact with you?"

> They spoke normally to me, "Oksana, come on," it was fine. They explained the episiotomy to me, that there was meconium in the fluid, and that was it. They saw it and had to hurry. But I have very mixed feelings about it all. On the one hand, I had no complaints about the payment. It was a wonderful room, with wonderful rugs, a big room with very pretty curtains, icons, a bed for me with pillows, a bed for my mother, a changing table. All the sheets were clean, they brought them in for the baby. So I can't complain about that. It was all fine.
>
> But on the other hand, emotionally, I was very dissatisfied. It was a case where you want something specific and are aiming for it, and your illusions are shattered. I know they were looking after the baby, since there was meconium in the fluid, but on the other hand, I thought that if they hadn't broken the water and I'd have given birth myself, the meconium would've come out during the birth, and they wouldn't have given me an episiotomy. I was terribly upset afterward; I cried and cried.

Oksana's dissatisfaction with the birth came from repeated experiences that her needs were ignored, displaced unnecessarily by a series of routinized medical interventions. She felt that the midwife's decision to break her water was entirely unjustified, but led to a further series of undesirable interventions, including getting the episiotomy and having the baby taken from her following the delivery, despite her clear desire to have him put on her stomach immediately. If Oksana understood at one level that the meconium in the fluid was a sign of danger to the baby, she had no clear sense of how and why it was serious, or what precisely the personnel did to protect the baby—she describes them as having cleansed him off and swaddled him, rather than undertaking procedures such as aspiration that would seem to have justified their decisions. Consequently, she felt that their discussion of the meconium provided an excuse to do things the way they wanted, to justify their continued dominance as professionals.

Feminist critics of medicalized models of birth in the West have emphasized that the introduction of a consumer model of childbirth has effectively displaced, rather than solved, critical concerns about the need to demedicalize birth (Davis-Floyd 1992). Oksana's case demonstrates that this had clearly been the case in Russia as well. She had hoped that accessing care through official channels and official payments would enable a new type of professional relationship with the staff, without the personal obligations inherent in acquaintance relations. She told of her desire for good conditions and "normal" interactions, and had no complaints about the aesthetic quality of the rooms or politeness of the personnel. But Oksana's payment had no affect on the medicalized character of birth; it gave her no authority in the birth process and left her expressed desires—to not be on the gynecological chair, to avoid an episiotomy, to have the baby immediately put to the breast—ignored.

INNA'S STORY

Inna was twenty-eight years old when she gave birth in June 1999. She had completed one of the newly opened secretarial schools in St. Petersburg and worked as an office manager for a private firm before having her first child. Her husband also held a midlevel position in a private company, with a moderately comfortable salary. Like Oksana's, Inna's story offers insights into the many aspects of women's interests that are not guaranteed by the new neoliberal service model. Inna delivered at a paid ward where she expected to be treated by an acquaintance-physician. She explicitly wanted a private room and an acquaintance-doctor, "because even if you pay, you still don't know who you're going to end up with." Still, she only found an acquaintance-physician two weeks before she gave birth. Her in-laws had connections to the medical field, and they were finally able to locate someone who knew someone who could help. She met with the doctor, and they agreed that Inna would be admitted to the prenatal ward on the Wednesday before she was due.

> But it was a hot summer, and I just refused to go. And the next day, it all started. So I called that woman who I had an arrangement with, and I don't know what was going on, but she says, "Unfortunately, I can't take you." I say to her, "What am I supposed to do?" And she says, "Well, you were planning to go to the paid ward, right?" Well, we were, for besides the fact that she herself was supposed to take part in it—I had already paid. They were monsters.
>
> The doctor says, "The only thing I can do for you, since I'm leaving to go to work at another hospital right now, is to arrange for you to have a room [on the paid ward]." We had made an arrangement and paid for everything.

"And how was the birth?"

Well, of course now it's scary to think about it, but at the time, nobody really knew anything. I mean, I was really happy that everything turned out so wonderfully. . . . I didn't even feel anything. Well, I felt something, of course, but very calmly and tolerable. I arrived at the hospital and was already half the way dilated (5 cm), had very little pain and felt fine.

Then, as they typically do in our hospitals, they decided to make it go faster. They gave me a shot to induce me. Naturally everything then got fairly intense. After a while the doctor examined me and said, "Well, it's strange but we've stimulated your labor and somehow, for some reason, the dilation has stopped, or, it didn't end, but slowed down." It was going much better when I arrived. She said to me, "Now it's fairly serious, and may actually be very serious, because we don't know exactly how much it's slowed down." But for me it's all going pretty intense. I got a little scared. . . . And then they say to me, "Let's give you a shot against the pain, it only costs $100."

Inna described these initial experiences as "typical" of the worst of Soviet maternity hospitals—the routine stimulation of labor, even when not medically indicated, and institutionally induced illness, or iatrogenesis, that results. It also reflected the worst side of a market logic—a readiness to commercialize any possible transaction, even demanding additional fees for pain relief from a birthing woman. But her negative experience continued. The anesthesia didn't work, and she overheard the doctors talking among themselves that this kind of injection was supposed to be administered early in labor, while she had erroneously been given it toward the end. Finally, they told Inna's husband to stay in the waiting room while they were giving her the anesthesia, and they never called him in again. He remained quietly waiting outside the delivery room, because, in Inna's words, "he's the obedient type. Moreover, at the clinic they warned us not to contradict the doctors, they know what they're doing and they don't like it when someone begins to demand their rights [*prava kachat'*]."

While neither Inna nor her husband "demanded their rights," Inna did make a request of the midwife to try and avoid an episiotomy:

I had read a book about birth and so I said to the midwife, "I know that there's this particular thing that's often done—in order to lighten the work load, they generally cut you. Please, you know, I don't have a big baby, he's really not big, he's just fine for me." I said, "Don't cut me, please, specially. I don't have a big baby, maybe I can do it myself. Just tell me at the time whether it's possible." And she got really insulted and said, "We never just cut people." And I was like, "Oh, well, maybe the author was mistaken, or I misheard."

"How did it work out?"

"It turned out quite simply that nobody had any time to do anything; it all ripped on its own (laughs). I remember in the first moments after the birth, I asked, 'Is there a cut?' And she says, 'No, no, nobody did anything.'"

While Inna luckily avoided the episiotomy, she felt that overall her care both had been negligent and had not been in accordance with the ward's own promises for a "family birth." When asked if she lodged a complaint afterward, Inna explained:

> It wasn't possible to. The thing is, there was a contract. We had read it from the beginning. They especially give it to you in the very beginning, when you just arrive. The thing is that there's this point [in the contract], well, to put it crudely, everything they do is justified. . . . They did it all wrong, they didn't call my husband back in. And so it turned out that there were no witnesses. So, if for example, I began to raise complaints that the anesthesia didn't work, well, who can prove that?

Although several medical interventions were blatant mistakes, and the offer of anesthesia for additional payment seemed unethical, Inna felt she had no rights to complain and seek compensation. If the neoliberal service model generated a language of comfort and attention, Inna's story reveals it did virtually nothing to transfer power to women over their birth experience. Consumers bought services, but had no political influence or social power to defend themselves. Introduced in select wings with attractive décor, the service model remained compatible with a broader system of medicalized childbirth, which did nothing to challenge warnings to women and their husbands not to question the doctors or demand their rights.

Given the lack of institutionalized legal rights for patients and adequate conditions to enforce them, the "guarantee" of safety and "all the best" was reduced to advertising rhetoric alone. Attractive conditions, polite staff attitudes, and even disposable needles and adequate supplies did nothing to empower women to understand the interventions being proposed, ensure their rights to participate in decision-making, and provide them channels for compensation in the case of error. The contract Inna signed was not mutually beneficial, but protected the institution. The service model served the needs of the hospital.

During my tour of St. Petersburg maternity hospitals in 1994, I asked one highly placed administrator whether his hospital would be establishing a ward with paid services. "We've been debating the idea," he said, but the organizational changes involved would be extensive and complicated, and the staff had not yet made a decision. Then with a warm smile, he added his own opinion of the trend toward paid maternity care: "Actually, *we* should probably be paying these women, rather than demanding that they pay us!"

For this doctor, women who gave birth were making a social contribution, one that deserved to be rewarded rather than made more difficult by economic obstacles. This was one of only a few comments I heard from providers that linked demographic concerns over the low birth rate to health care policies. Instead, the frenetic pace of economic stratification and impoverishment created under neoliberal reforms led most providers to look inward at their own pocketbooks as they considered necessary paths for restructuring women's health care. As we have seen, the legitimation of monetary exchange occurred in several ways: in an institutional focus on establishing fee-for-service care as the single most important maternity care reform of the decade; in providers' gradual acceptance of monetary payments as compatible with, and even necessary for, professional integrity—even when exchanged unofficially; and in patients' growing sense that paying money (usually to acquaintance-doctors) was the key to securing improved care. The stories of Masha, Oksana, and Inna further demonstrate a curious phenomenon in their diverse approaches to paid services. When considering their own strategies of ensuring improved care, all of these women focused their attention on the personal, internal qualities of the providers they dealt with. Masha's views were the most conventional in terms of long-standing Russian notions of money. When she stated that accessing paid care was less important than the need for an acquaintance-physician who would ensure quality treatment, she subtly suggested that money was not a prime vehicle for change. Indeed, throughout her narrative, she portrayed the staff of the paid ward as totally disinterested in money, and claimed that their altruistic concern for their work was what distinguished them from staff on the free ward and staff from paying wards in other hospitals. For Masha, the individual characteristics of caregivers were the single most important factor in determining the quality of care she could expect—and structural issues such as the salaries they earned, the conditions of their work, and the types of work they did (such as ironing in every free moment) would have no affect on those who were truly committed professionals. She echoed the sentiment presented above by Leva, who saw money as deeply distasteful and people who valued wealth as morally suspicious (cf. Ries 1997). Yet even while Masha construed monetary payments as an inappropriate focus for defining personal and professional legitimacy, she envisioned social change based on individualized character development rather than recognizing structural needs for reform.

Inna sought to have the assistance of an acquaintance-doctor to ensure the provider's personal concern for her care. Her story reveals how unreliable the use of informal relations was to secure women's needs. First, her acquaintance-doctor failed to follow through on their agreement and left her to give birth anonymously with the paid ward staff. Then, without any formal procedures for petitioning for her needs, such as avoiding an episiotomy, she tried to negotiate informally with the midwife to avoid it. Finally, despite the fact that the staff failed to fulfill their promises of having her husband at the birth and her sense that several interventions were blatant cases of medical error, she had no structured rights to complain and seek compensation. Monetary payment offered more attractive and spacious conditions while in the hospital, but had no positive effect on her rights as a patient.

Oksana experienced the same outcome. She sought paid births both for the luxurious conditions they would provide and to avoid the personal kinds of dependency that accompany acquaintance-based favors. She was one of several women I met who explicitly articulated the notion that paying for services would establish new forms of professional relationships—what she called "normal" relations. Interestingly, my friend Valia, a successful businesswoman, expressed a very similar vision to Oksana's. When I first asked Valia how she felt about paying for medical services, and whether it was a moral thing to do, she replied without hesitation, "Oh, definitely. We have to get over that Soviet nonsense [*sovetskie zamorochki*] that people should work for free. I feel that I *should* pay, I have the money, and so it's right that I pay for their professionalism and time."

With such comments, Valia and Oksana defined paying for health care as a moral action that conveyed recognition and respect for the professional's attention and expertise. By personally accepting an obligation to pay for a doctor's time and skills, they saw themselves transcending Soviet-era taboos regarding money. Oksana contrasted "modern," professional women doctors, who take money for their work, with old-style Soviet doctors, who worked "for free" and behaved with "impudence" [*khamstvo*]. Instead of impudence, authoritarianism, and rudeness, Oksana explained, "modern" professionals interacted in "normal" ways—they were friendly and cognizant of the need to provide "clients" with attentive "service" [*servis*]. Yet neither Valia's nor Oksana's payments accessed for them the systemic rights and personal empowerment they felt were absolutely necessary for ensuring good treatment and positive experiences. Both critically concluded that if they give birth again, they would travel abroad. "Only in Finland," Oksana swore to me, never again in Russia.

* * *

The notion that competition leads to improved quality care has been challenged by numerous studies in the U.S. and Europe that show how the drive to earn profits in health care can easily work against patient interests (Light 2000). In Russia, this possibility has been taken to the extreme, for the ideological celebration of profitability has occurred without concomitant changes in political, economic, and legal systems to protect laypersons. Medical procedures that often become the center of conflict between women and providers, such as the routine use of episiotomies, remain unaddressed, leaving this an arena replete with tension in actual practice. Nor did a market logic for health services ameliorate most of the basic structural problems in the organization of health care. It did not establish continuity of care for women's health; if individual women now had the theoretical right to buy prenatal consultations with the doctor who would attend them at birth, the overall system of maternity care was not changed. Prenatal care continued to be structurally separated from birth and postpartum care, all of which were divided from general adult health services. Many women arranged unofficial agreements with providers of their choice to obtain some continuity of care; the poorest and most marginalized women, unable to forge official or unofficial agreements, continued to bear the brunt of a structurally divided system.

What the legalization and spread of fee-for-service maternity care did do was to transform childbirth into a consumer service. Hospitals now offered women the opportunity to buy more comfortable conditions, privacy, and access to their personal support system with companions during and after birth. Certainly, these were positive developments that have helped to make childbirth a less isolating and uncomfortable event for some women. Yet competition did not work in any simple way to the benefit of consumers. Competition led organizations to elaborate their offerings and thereby create a set of desires, by presenting to the public the kinds of needs and interests they have regarding expert care in childbirth. Thus, hospitals distinguished paid services from the basic level of care offered to all residents for "free," by creating "hotel-like" luxury conditions, including private rooms with bathrooms and attractive decor. Comfort, decor, politeness, and technological superiority were the main products for sale. By contrast, other possible needs of birthing women, such as being involved in clinical decisions, were not acknowledged. Moreover, these discoveries set the ideological parameters of "responsibility" at the level of the individual, rather than conceptualizing collective rights and institutional responsibilities as well. At the same time, with neither consumer watchdog groups nor governmental regulation on fee-for-service care, women remained rather vulnerable to both provider domination and financial exploitation by institutions focusing on making a profit.

While promising "professionalism," including the staff's "timely attention and proper attitude," these hospitals worked to maintain expert dominance over the birthing experience and ensure patient compliance. Positioning the medical expert as "service provider" and the patient as "consumer" enabled hospitals to define as most important those elements of childbirth that were largely unrelated to the actual medical interventions, despite portraying their offerings as better quality care. Competition enhanced the power of institutions by generating a language of newness and quality guarantees—of "service"—while obscuring the continuing lack of legal protections and rights that characterized the Soviet system. The service model changed the kind of care women get in birth, mainly by ensuring that their medicalized subordination could be carried out in privacy.

Questioning the virtue of a market orientation for health care, sociologists committed to issues of equity have developed a moral framework for evaluating health care delivery and financing systems that is broadly relevant for either a state or market model. Ten "benchmarks of fairness" (Caplan, Light, and Daniels 1999: 858) seem especially pertinent for imagining the kinds of regulations that would need to be in place to address equity and fairness:

1. Universal access in coverage, including full portability and continuity;
2. Universal access regarding nonfinancial barriers such as language, culture, information, and class;
3. Comprehensive and uniform benefits;
4. Equitable financing with community-rated contributions and minimum discrimination via cash payments.
5. Equitable financing in which all direct and indirect out-of-pocket expenses are scaled to household budget and ability to pay.
6. Value for money through clinical efficiency, with a focus on primary care, public health and prevention, and the minimization of both overutilization and underutilization;
7. Value for money through systemic efficiency, by minimizing administrative overhead and cost shifting, tough contractual bargaining, and anti-fraud and abuse measures;
8. Public accountability through explicit, public, and detailed procedures for evaluating services, with full, public reports; explicit, democratic procedures for allocation decisions; fair grievances procedures; adequate privacy protection;
9. Comparability between health care budget and other programs;
10. Informed consumer choice regarding primary care providers, specialists, other providers, and procedures.

Whether in a state-controlled, nonprofit, or market-based system, working to achieve these criteria would require well-funded, organized state regulatory bodies, consumer protection groups, and mechanisms for enforcement of fairness criteria.

Finally, it is necessary to consider moral criteria of fairness for health care providers, too. Empowering physicians in the post-Soviet era through a profit-oriented competitive model that rewards an economic logic for clinical decisions has the potential to damages the ethics of physicians as well as the health of users. Creating an "incentive" system for providers *to the exclusion of a basic living wage* treats providers as mechanistic robots who are expected to "respond" to no other political and social empowerment than financial carrots. It rewards economic considerations over compassion, professional pride, and dedication to healing. When health system reformers narrowly addressed providers' interests through facilitating competition and profitability, they virtually excluded Russian providers from public policy. Providers' voices remain widely silenced.

Conclusion

TRANSFORMING FEMINIST STRATEGIES

The global and local efforts to solve Russia's reproductive health crisis shared an intriguing set of tactics: all worked to bypass the state and public sphere as the primary site for change, and created imperatives for moral work on the self and interpersonal relations. From WHO's maternal health project to Russian public health reforms, to local sex education classes and provider-patient negotiations, actors placed their hope in individualized, personalized, and privatized kinds of development, rather than prioritizing changes in institutions and changes for the benefit of collectivities. If policymakers justified this approach as disciplining individuals to take personal responsibility after living for generations under Soviet paternalism, ordinary citizens and health providers tended to regard the state with utter distrust; their strategies were marked by a thorough resignation to the fact that formal institutions and procedures would simply not become sources of justice or social protection.

We have seen, also, that the emphasis on individualized, personalized, and privatized types of change has stemmed from a variety of sources. From its inception, the Soviet state created imperatives for individual citizens to adopt new morals suited to the demands of a collective society (Field 1996; Kharkhordin 1999; Sinyavsky 1990; Volkov 2000). Traces of Soviet didacticism remained evident in health care services in the 1990s, as when physicians blamed poor public health indicators and social problems on women themselves and when gynecologist-educators threatened that people's physical and emotional health depended on their willingness to adhere to proper sexual and reproductive behavior, while almost never acknowledging the broader influences of socioeconomic factors. People's responses to such discourses have varied over time and space. Doctors and women patients, for example, reproduced aspects of Soviet ideology by endorsing the need for raising individuals' "levels of *kul'turnost'*," by explaining the inadequacies of health care services or pregnancy/birth outcomes as stemming from a lack of "personal responsibility," and by strategizing to "take responsibility" for themselves, rather than struggling for political, economic, and institutional forms of change. As we have seen, these discourses and strategies also dovetailed closely with the neoliberal imperatives of global and Russian health policymakers to stimulate new, "dynamic" modes of interaction and personality traits. On the other hand, doctors and patients also opposed state imperatives, as when they resisted connecting personal decisions about childbearing to national demographic needs.

Much research has documented the salient cultural dichotomy between personal and collectivist interests and the long-standing value Russians have placed on personal spheres of life and relationships, as opposed to public and formal ones (Boym 1994; Dunham 1990; Field 1996; Tolstaya 1990). Ledeneva has connected such concerns to create moral interpersonal interactions with the "economy of favors" so central to Soviet society (Ledeneva 1998). This study builds on Ledeneva's findings by showing how the reliance on informal, personalizing tactics in the health sphere emerged as a response to the state's ongoing failures to fulfill its promise to ensure adequate level of health services. If evading official procedures through arrangements based on personal connections was central to the socialist system's very functioning (Verdery 1996), "democratic" reforms have done little to make such practices anachronistic in the realm of health care. While Russia's new compulsory medical insurance system officially claimed to guarantee all maternity care free of charge, it did not supply sufficient funding for basic medicines and equipment for births.[1] Deploying informal strategies to manage such regularly occurring contradictions and constraints thus continued to serve as a coping strategy for Russian doctors and patients in the first decade of neoliberal reforms. But rather than viewing these practices as signs of persistent (or new forms of) "corruption," I have stressed that under ongoing conditions of systemic hindrance and hypocrisy, informal practices often aimed to fulfill moral obligations to others. Unofficial payments for maternity care offer a prime example. Many patients feared that paying for services through official channels would do little to improve their doctors' personal economic well-being; negotiating private, informal arrangements gave women both greater hope that their doctor would be personally committed to their care, and seemed an ethically appropriate way of overcoming the injustices health workers faced in the unfair payment system hospital administrators had devised. It is evident from these cases that both Soviet experiences and neoliberal reforms have shaped the current logic of locating social change at the level of individual morality and of pursuing social transformations through informal and privatizing tactics. Similarly, they have both ensured the ongoing invisibility of gender as an issue related to social inequality.

The challenge of reconciling feminist ideals of gender equality, social justice, and community empowerment with local Russian knowledge and practice has been a primary inspiration for this inquiry. I opened the ethnography with two driving questions: why did Russian health experts reject the ideology of women's self-determination in health care, and what solutions did they and others—including women patients—pursue instead for resolving Russia's crisis in reproduction? Exploring local projects and practices ethnographically raised important insights into the range of solutions desired by groups located in distinct socioeconomic spaces. We have seen how women with financial means chose to use new, paid maternity services or even planned to go abroad; women with both economic and social resources strove to pay *acquaintance*-physicians, while the poorest and most socially vulnerable women relied on free public services and sought to "take responsibility" for themselves, often maintaining deep distrust in doctors' recommendations. Despite such differences, however, women from all economic backgrounds, and health experts, shared a sensibility that relying on the state and public sphere for social justice or practical assistance was futile, and that healing—both individuals and society as a whole—required concerted efforts to cultivate personal strengths, morals, and interpersonal relations. The imperative to "change yourself, and the whole world will change around you" resonated with health educators and policy reformers, clinic providers and patients—despite the diverse and sometimes contradictory thrusts of their health-related endeavors.

Clearly, such cultural logics pose striking challenges for feminist observers committed to the struggle against *social* inequities. What strategies can we effectively and ethically pursue that are both culturally meaningful and in tune with critical feminist agendas in this post-socialist, neoliberal moment? How can we promote a reform agenda that realizes the most radical of democratic promises for broad-based opportunities, recognizes the social nature of interests, and maintains a concern with marginalized sectors of society? One solution is to serve as insistent, critical observers of the neoliberal privatizing policies advocated by global and local elites, highlighting their uneven, often unjust effects, and provocatively exposing their failures to achieve their self-proclaimed goals of increasing prosperity (Scheper-Hughes 1990). The cases in this book have shown that personal and privatizing strategies repeatedly produced less than actors hoped: doctors' efforts to resist the "collective irresponsibility" structured into the health care system through individual, heroic efforts of taking "personal responsibility" for their work were unable to overcome the range of obstacles stemming from poverty, political disenfranchisement, and the fragmented nature of the system itself. Patients' tactics of accessing maternity care through acquaintances also usually failed to overcome these structural constraints, and fell short of providing them with the caring, competent attention they needed. The privatizing policy of introducing market mechanisms without state and nongovernmental oversight raised new compromises for patient care. The haphazard establishment of fee-for-service births outside a living wage for health providers increased both conflicts between providers themselves and the likelihood that providers would increasingly expect underground payments. By highlighting these processes, I hope to introduce a critical analysis of privatizing, individualizing policies and practices in the health care sphere in order to widen debate about possible alternative methods of improving the health care system for patients and providers alike.

In no small part, this argument is directed at international organizations and activists. I have suggested that global assistance projects must adopt a critical stance toward governmentality, first and foremost by acknowledging the losses Russians have suffered through particular global and state policies, such as the destruction of social rights that has been central to neoliberalism. This contrasts with the tactics WHO consultants deployed during their training workshop on empowering women in birth, when they insisted to providers, "You can't change the government, but you can change what you do everyday." While the need to instrumentalize feminist goals inevitably requires addressing only a select range of social inequities in any given project, we must not allow our own bureaucratically imposed limitations to blind us to the larger experiences shaping the lives of the people we purport to be helping.

The goal of realizing new ways to pursue feminist critiques and struggles has been one of the most important contributions of scholarship concerned with gender issues in the aftermath of socialism (Funk and Mueller 1993; Gal and Kligman 2000a, b). Gal and Kligman's path-breaking findings that the political transformations of Eastern European states since 1989 have been thoroughly imbued with gendered inequalities—from the drastic reduction in women's political participation to the reconfiguration of gendered, public-private splits in social spheres, to the centrality of anti-abortion policies in every state except Romania—confirm that gender is no peripheral matter in the business of state and nation building. It is structured at the very core of the political process (Gal and Kligman 2000a).

Inspired by such work, my goal has nonetheless been somewhat distinct: I have underscored the workings of "reproductive politics" at the local level of clinic reforms and provider-patient relations. This lens, I believe, has brought into focus important dimensions of the daily work of creating social change, including the ways that people's strategies respond to and confirm policy thrusts aiming to absolve the state from ensuring workers' and citizens' basic needs. Yet my concern with highlighting local knowledge and practices for the sake of revitalizing feminist activism also requires attending to the political campaigns surrounding reproductive issues in Russia. For it is in the work of pro-natalist activists, ironically, that we find the most avid willingness to pursue political activity in the name of collective needs. Three groups of pro-natalists have been most active in Russia, and their discourses for collective needs enjoy moral legitimacy.

A COLLECTIVE POLITICS FOR REPRODUCTION: PRO-NATALISM

Not surprisingly, pro-natalists' agenda in reproduction has been less focused on ensuring general improvements in women's health than on increasing childbearing productivity. Their ranks were filled largely with professionals, such as demographers, sociologists, educators, and church officials; their prolific, rhetorically skillful writings fill the academic and popular presses with cries for urgent policy measures aimed at rescuing the Russian nation from imminent "extinction." Pro-natalist activities also included holding conferences, sitting on government committees, and collecting petitions to lobby government officials to stop the "destruction" of the family. While Russian providers and women repeatedly told me that collective action for improving women's health would be unfeasible and/ or spiritually tainting, pro-natalists portrayed their work in lobbying the state and entering the public sphere as heroic steps to save the nation, and even the world, from its current paths of self-destruction (Antonov and Sorokin 2002).

Pro-natalists followed distinct political platforms. Generally speaking, they included communists, anti-communists, and religious nationalists. Pro-natalist policies tended to be supported by health professionals, who sometimes discussed the "dying out of the nation" in the press but were not as active as these other groups. The political differences between these groups affected their attitudes toward both the Soviet past and the kinds of policies they advocated for increasing fertility rates. For example, communists have depicted "the death of the nation" as a direct outcome of the poverty resulting from market reforms. They advocated reversing demographic decline through a return to economic planning and a strong paternalist welfare state (Khorev 1995, 1997). In focusing on Russia's current devastating poverty, communists compared the advent of market reforms with the ravages of war, bombings, and plague. One demographer and communist supporter characterized the falling population as a "demographic Chernobyl" (Khorev 1997). Linking demographic decline with national "extinction," the Communist Party of the Russian Federation introduced impeachment proceedings against Boris Yeltsin, in part for perpetuating the "genocide of the Russian people" through his economic reforms.

Anti-communist pro-natalists have advocated different types of policies for increasing the birth rate. One of the most prolific scholars of fertility decline since the early 1980s, Moscow University sociology professor Anatolii Antonov, has linked decreased childbearing to the "breakdown of family values" occurring throughout the world since the mid twentieth century. In the Soviet Union, he asserted, this problem was exacerbated by the forced inclusion of women in the labor force, which supposedly decreased their interest in mothering. Soviet socialist policies on women's "equality" hastened the demise of the Russian family and nation, Antonov contended, and the most necessary measures to reverse these trends should focus on raising the value of family life for society.[2] Families needed to reject selfish interests in consumerism and embrace childbearing and family life for their own good and the good of the nation. Unlike the communists', the policies Antonov advocated to ensure this change focus on supporting the development of family-based businesses as a new structural organization benefiting both families and the state. Family businesses, he argued, offer an acceptable, privatizing alternative to Soviet paternalism, with the additional advantage of making individuals' economic prosperity dependent on family life. Such a policy both reversed Soviet policies of state-based employment, which ensured women's economic independence from men, and combated the perceived individualism of current market reforms, which Antonov saw as buttressing the authority of each individual person over that of the family as a whole. Thus, despite his partial support of privatizing economic patterns, Antonov clearly placed collective, national needs over personal interests. "Individual choice," Antonov argued, must not be allowed to overtake the demographic and social needs of society for strong, nuclear families (headed by men) that ensure moderate population growth (Antonov and Sorokin 2002: 32).

A third coalition of nationalists and religious activists has also worked to revive the traditional, patriarchal family and oppose women's autonomy. Throughout the 1990s, they took aim at Russia's fledgling family planning and sex education initiatives, accusing organizations involved in promoting birth control of working strategically to accelerate Russia's depopulation. Merging pro-natalism with nationalism and anti-Western sentiment, they have depicted sex education and family planning as foreign perversions designed to warp Russian youth psychologically and brainwash them to despise family life (Babasyan 1995; Medvedeva and Shishova 2000; Molodsova 1999).

Such efforts succeeded in August 2003, when the Russian Ministry of Health severely curtailed the criteria through which Russian women could access abortion in the second trimester. These coalitions have also had direct effects on the work of the Russian Family Planning Association. In the spring of 1997, Russia's anti-abortion organizations and a public committee called "For the Moral Regeneration of the Fatherland" sponsored by the Russian Orthodox Church, working in collaboration with the nationalist activists, submitted to the Duma batches of signed petitions asking the government to rescind funding for family planning. The Duma made the topic the subject of a roundtable discussion on "Family Planning in the Context of Russia's National Security" and consequently voted to end funding of its presidential family planning program that had been established in the early 1990s (Babasyan 1999). On the legislative front, Church organizers were instrumental in promoting a 1997 draft law that would have made abortion illegal in all but medically indicated cases (Bateneva 1997). The restrictions on second trimester abortion appear to be only the first successful legislative achievement in what is undoubtedly a long-term campaign to link childbearing to the nation's survival and entangle anti-Western sentiment with opposition to family planning.

These groups' tactics have exploited the public's lack of awareness of the legislative process and general alienation from policymaking. For example, in draft laws they introduced to restrict women's access to abortion, they tended to do so surreptitiously by burying the abortion issue within broader legislation concerning "bioethics" or "protection of mothers and children" (Ballaeva 1998; Bateneva 1998). This language has seeped into the discourses of other groups, including some health professionals, who have written about the need for policy measures to preserve the Russian "gene pool" (*Delovoi Peterburg* 2000: 9). By connecting pro-natalist activism and "bioethical" debates with the revitalization of the "Fatherland," "Russia's national security," and "the protection of mothers and children," nationalists have aligned themselves with morally legitimate forms of collective interests (Gal and Kligman 2000a). Even more alarming, following the Ministry of Health's decision in August 2003 to restrict abortion access, there was very little press coverage of the new policy (U.S. and British newspapers, by contrast, covered the change rather widely). Several Russian professionals I spoke with in the fall of 2003 knew nothing about the new regulations. The concrete dismantlement of abortion access, it seems, is occurring through creeping administrative policies that preclude public debate, just as women and men's needs for ensuring safe, timely conceptions almost never emerge in pro-natalist discussions.

Pro-natalists' hostility to family planning efforts is ironic, because organizations and practitioners of Russia's reproductive health establishment see themselves devotedly working to ensuring women's capabilities to successfully bear children, to promote the moral revitalization of traditional families, and to support the nation's future vitality, as the content of their sex education and family planning projects revealed. Many Russian reproductive health clinics received financial and moral support from Western anti-abortion organizations for their work against abortion. None of the institutions providing abortions wanted to suggest—either tacitly or explicitly—that it promotes or morally sanctions the use of abortion. Even those Russian organizations with ties to the global reproductive rights movement did not publicly advertise the issue of reproductive "rights." When the Russian Family Planning Association was established in 1992 as a branch of the nongovernmental International Federation of Planned Parenthood, it received the blessing of the Yeltsin administration for its contribution to reducing the number of abortions and resolving the country's demographic crisis. It has drawn from its international parent movement in discussing the need for "safe motherhood" and "reproductive health," and it occasionally invokes a language of "freedom" and "rights"; but Russian family planning advocates have largely contextualized their activity in terms of Russia's particular needs to lower the abortion rate by providing safe contraceptive alternatives. As we saw, activists who initiated sex education programs for Russian school children and teenagers conceptualized their cause as strengthening reproductive health and family life. Such projects were initiated by doctors and psychologists who with great concern confronted sharply rising rates of pregnancy and sexually transmitted disease among teens. They, too, have often cooperated with global anti-abortion proponents, described in the web sites of organizations such as Human Life International (Human Life International 2001). Collective needs, in these cases, tend to be construed in terms of the moral—spiritual—character of the society and nation. Or, as we saw in the lectures by obstetrician-educator Anastasia Pavlovna, discourses describing the fetus as an individual *"lichnost'"* can be deployed to underscore women's responsibilities to others—in this case, their children and families.

TRANSFORMING FEMINIST STRATEGIES

Amidst these vibrant political campaigns, there has not been a substantial, mass response against pro-natalism by Russian women. Newly formed Russian women's groups, while supporting the concept of reproductive rights, have focused the majority of their activism and research on problems of women's economic survival (Bridger, Kay, and Pinnick 1996: 119, 166; Hemment 2000, 2004a, b; Moscow Center for Gender Studies

2001; Sperling 1999; but see Ballaeva 1998 as one exception). There are complex reasons for the absence of feminist opposition to pro-natalism. First and foremost, the overwhelming consensus that Russia is facing a severe demographic crisis threatening the nation's very existence has made it exceedingly difficult to combat pro-natalist efforts on the basis of "women's right to choose." Such arguments would appear to value the interests of women over those of the nation as a whole, leaving feminist discourses vulnerable to charges of "selfishness" and indifference to the fate of the nation. Closely connected to this is the value of "family" in Russian public discourse, on the one hand, and the negative images associated with feminism as breeding animosity to family life and men, on the other. Throughout the Soviet era, the "family" and domestic sphere figured into local strategies of resistance to socialist ideology on collectivism, as well as to the everyday, symbolic violence of bureaucratic indifference. Russian women and men (as their counterparts in Eastern Europe), privileged family as the moral, personal "refuge" from official spheres, and considered it an arena outside of state power (Funk 1993; Havelkova 1993; Tolstaya 1990; Toth 1993). Feminism, by contrast, has been largely construed in the Russian media as a hostile movement of socially alienated, deviant women, motivated only by self-interest and a perverse desire to destroy the family. Pro-natalists have directly contributed to these images, and have expanded them to include attacks against gay rights organizations, supporters of alternative family forms, and single mothers (e.g., Antonov and Sorokin 2002).[3]

In this context of widespread hostility against discourses prioritizing women's interests in reproduction, on the one hand, and the privatization of agency occurring in public health contexts, on the other, feminist concerns to improve women's health, autonomy, and equality face formidable challenges. A key intervention of this ethnography has been to bring local Russian knowledge and practices to the center of feminist attention, to help readers concerned with enhancing democratizing changes to understand the logics behind Russian efforts in reproductive health. In reflecting on the projects and practices I observed throughout this research, I have concluded that feminist activists would benefit from adopting two key strategies in their work in Russia—and, undoubtedly, in other global sites as well.

First, it is necessary to find a mode of advocating for women's interests that is compatible with Russian concerns with personal morality and interpersonal obligation, and to diminish images of feminism as hostile to families. Admittedly, this represents a difficult and potentially uncomfortable move, inasmuch as normative kinds of discourses have, for good reason, been considered highly suspect in critical feminist struggles. And still, it may be time to investigate alternative possibilities to the liberal individualism central to much American feminism.[4] Widespread images of feminists as alienated, anti-family, and selfishly individualistic have long enjoyed hegemony in Russia and elsewhere; in many post-socialist contexts, this image has successfully marginalized feminist discourse so extensively that it has not been able to gain a foothold in the public consciousness.[5] It is notable that those discourses promoting "individualism" in public health reforms, sex education projects, and the informal strategies between providers and patients do not overlap neatly with the kind of individualism found in American liberal thought. Rather, these projects and practices promoted a concern with privatizing strategies and "individualism" that unambiguously aimed to enhance people's ethical standards and interpersonal obligations. Health reformers, for example, believed that competition would stimulate providers to improve their skills and provide better services to patients (not merely to work out of the self-interest of enhancing their own salaries); educators striving to cultivate a sense of individual *lichnost'* did so in order to promote healthier sexual relations and, ultimately, more satisfying and successful marriages; and patients and providers each argued for the need for increased individual *responsibility* in health practices and work ethics, not for a renewed focus on individualism in a utilitarian or self-interested way, or a platform of individual rights.

I believe that a more promising strategy for feminist activists in Russia would strive to promote an ethics of societal responsibility, a concern with collective obligations toward caregiving, rather than highlighting a concern with individual rights and autonomy (Tronto 1993). Such discourses could challenge neoliberal policies in the post-socialist context on the basis that they do not enhance people's welfare, but harm the well-being of vulnerable groups, including women, children, and working-class men. Moreover, it is necessary to highlight how even those with great financial resources suffer when the need for competition gets prioritized above safety and personal needs—as the case of paid maternity care demonstrated. Feminists could acknowledge local concerns with high morbidity to underscore the growing problems of caring for disabled people and to highlight how women and men, mothers and fathers, need social supports and resources to allow their children (and each other) to reach their greatest possible potential. These discourses would, furthermore, enable feminists to tap into Russian concerns with promoting the "spiritual" wholeness of people (meant here in the sense not of religious doctrine but of psycho-social harmony, the emotional health of individuals and building of communities). In other words, I argue that it is necessary to adapt feminist politics to local idioms, even highlighting selective kinds of issues that may be more easily defended, over those that seem most important in our own contexts.

For example, rather than to focus on defending women's rights to abortion or autonomy in birth, a more viable strategy of promoting women's health issues may be to focus on enabling women to take care of their health, preserve their ability to reproduce in safe and timely ways, and fulfill their and their family's needs most effectively. This has been a main thrust of the Russian Family Planning Association.[6] While such an approach may raise objections for running the risk of ignoring the fundamental issue of rights, I suggest that it represents an important, incremental, pragmatic step that takes the ideological context of Russia seriously. Such an approach would, moreover, offer an alternative to provider-educators who find themselves disinclined to blame sexually active teenagers, while still guarding against an "anything goes" mentality (Rivkin-Fish in press). Additionally, this kind of discourse would enable projects to address the interests of the highly feminized medical profession. Although an alliance with the medical profession may seem anathema to feminist critics of biomedicine, supporting the development of active professional associations with genuine influence on policymaking may be a key step in redirecting medical power away from the clinic and into the public sphere —provided that similarly influential health care users' groups are also organized and active. At a more basic level, critiques of neoliberalism could examine how doctors have been kept from satisfactorily achieving their work in healing and caregiving, and projects could address the collective disenfranchisement of doctors and patients as matters related to social vulnerability and poor health. We need innovative ways of ensuring both that people are not forced to take responsibility for themselves because they are abandoned by the health care and social welfare systems and that they have the means of becoming active participants in the health care process. If feminist projects take on this critique, come to be associated with an ethic of sympathy for the weakest and most vulnerable sectors of society, and offer concrete means for increasing interpersonal understanding and care, they will likely find wider acceptance among those invested in the healing professions as well as those seeking health care services.

A second strategy I propose for feminist activists and organizations working in the former Soviet world involves the need to examine and build on local initiatives for change that can serve as models for other local efforts. Adopting this strategy requires working in ways more compatible with anthropological approaches to research than has been done to date. For example, when WHO consultants working in St. Petersburg conducted a needs assessment study of Russian maternity services, they limited their investigations to official institutions and representatives accessed through the Public Health Committee. When I offered to introduce consultants to activists working in other sites and to establish informal meetings with Russians outside these official settings, the consultants refused, stating that they did not want to go beyond the mandate of their formal grant or develop additional obligations to people (Rivkin-Fish 2004b). Yet in the early 1990s, a range of activities was being initiated in St. Petersburg that aimed to realize innovations in women's health—some of which dovetailed with WHO's own values and goals. One important example was the burgeoning interest in homebirths. This unofficial, grass-roots movement worked semi-legally, facing deep suspicion among health providers in the official health care system, but rarely legal prosecution. Over the decade, homebirth midwives succeeded in organizing themselves into distinct schools and creating private practices, including an impressive childbirth education system attended by hundreds of St. Petersburg residents. One group of homebirth midwives I met and observed created a formal structure of costs and services for their clients (consciously refusing to label pregnant and birthing women as "patients" [*bol'nye*]). Had WHO consultants agreed to an anthropological type of inquiry that pursued the variety of local logics and practices for change, they could have turned their efforts to supporting such fledgling groups and then tapped into their culturally resonant discourses to render the arguments for demedicalization more in tune with Russian sensibilities.

In Russia, policies for structural adjustment, privatization, and withdrawing the state from social welfare provisions have, ironically, both been criticized for the severe poverty and vulnerability left in their wake and received ideological support from the numerous sectors of Russia's population who believe that the revitalization of society requires increasing "personal responsibility" and a certain sense of individualism. In daily life, these two positions have not necessarily been opposed to each other or been seen as mutually exclusive, for, as described above, doctors and patients tended to deploy both sets of arguments. Yet in the political sphere, these positions tend to be presented as mutually exclusive. While Russian communists stand at one extreme, bashing the market and seeking a return to Soviet-era controls, liberals occupy the other extreme, defending privatization with little interest in investigating the losses associated with market reforms.[7] Feminist organizations need to offer a middle ground that insists on addressing the interests of the poor and marginalized women and men, while also enabling the diversification of social institutions, discourses, and services facilitated by a nongovernmental, private sphere. Without returning to state paternalism, it is essential to make the state accountable for providing a reasonable safety net for residents, for fulfilling its obligations to fund the compulsory medical insurance system, and for ensuring health providers a living wage. Feminists involved in international agencies and development-based assistance need to advocate state regulation and oversight, as well as to support the development of consumer-based health groups to act as nongovernmental watchdogs.[8] This book, moreover, has shown the complex reasons that women in Russia have connected authoritative knowledge in biomedicine with personal relations (or even based the authority of medical expertise on cultural knowledge of providers' apparent "modernity," altruism, or impressions of a hospital's décor). Building on such findings, we may work to expand women's understandings of the very concept of medicalization, making the case that overcoming provider dominance can occur only with ideological, institutional, and legal transformations. By recognizing that demands for individual moral change have pushed away claims for social, economic, and institutional justice, feminists can position ourselves as critical activists struggling against structural violence (Farmer 1999). Finally, we must engage seriously and sincerely with local activists and ordinary Russian people. This involves approaching the project of "assistance" or "democracy" as an active, mutual exchange of ideas and insights, not a "training" project or a "mentoring" program. We must become willing to reform our systems of development—to democratize our politics of intervention.

NOTES

INTRODUCTION

1. Diagnosed cases of active tuberculosis, for example, increased 2.2 times between 1991 and 1998, reaching a rate of 76 cases per 100,000 population (in comparison with U.S. rates of approximately 10 per 100,000); sexually transmitted diseases (STDs) rose astronomically, with syphilis reaching a rate of 277.6 per 100,000 population in 1997, an increase of 64.5 times since 1989 (Vishnevskii 2000: 85–86).

Children and adolescents have seen significant rises in morbidity as well; cancer in this demographic age group, for example, rose 2.9 times between 1991 and 1998, and diseases related to the endocrine system, digestive system, and immune system rose 3.9 times in the same period (ibid., 90).

2. Besides WHO, a few such organizations included USAID, the Canadian International Development Association, Doctors without Borders, International Planned Parenthood Federation, and the Sexuality Information and Education Council of the US (SIECUS).

3. Hemment (2000, 2004a, b) and Sperling (1999), however, both show how most women's groups, working within the historical logics and economic constraints of post-socialism, have developed paths of civic engagement that differ dramatically from those of second-wave feminists in the West.

4. All names used in this book are pseudonyms, in accordance with anthropological conventions for protecting subjects' anonymity.

5. See, for example, Berdahl, Bunzl, and Lampland 2000; Buchowski 2001; Burawoy and Verdery 1999; Hann and Dunn 1996; Kennedy 2002; Verdery 1996, 1998 .

6. Burawoy, Krotov, and Lytkina 2000; Dunn 1999, 2004; Verdery 1996.

7. For more information on the World Health Organization and the European Regional Branch's Healthy Cities Project, see WHO's web site, www.who.dk/about who, and www.who.dk/healthy-cities, retrieved June 14, 2004.

8. Breastfeeding practices did not become a central focus of this study. During fieldwork, however, I did note that women's common practice of staying home during the months after giving birth facilitated breastfeeding during this initial period. However, the lack of social support resources for nursing, the lack of specialized breastfeeding clothes, and the need some women have for returning to work made breastfeeding for an entire year very difficult for most Russians.

9. Providers encouraged women to admit themselves to the hospital prior to labor in order to "prepare" physically for the birth. A factor women took into consideration in agreeing to do so is that the numerous drawbridges connecting parts of St. Petersburg open up each night between 2 A.M. and 6 A.M., making transportation between them impossible. If you lived on the other side of a bridge from your desired maternity hospital and labor began during the night, you might be forced to go to another hospital.

10. I undertook such "participant-conversations," usually lasting between thirty minutes and one hour, with forty-nine women in the hospital and with fifty-seven providers. I

conducted individual interviews with twenty-seven women, sixteen providers, and seven policymakers, and extended discussions about my research on more than one occasion with fourteen women, ten providers, and six policymakers from these "interview" groups, and in the process developed long-term friendships with many of them.

11. This rate was approximately seven times higher than in the U.S. and Great Britain.

12. See Comaroff 1982, 1985; Good 1994; Kleinman 1988, 1997, 1999; Kleinman, Das, and Lock 1997; Sargeant and Johnson 1996.

13. Das et al. 2001; Farmer 1992, 1999; Kleinman 1973; Kleinman, Das, and Lock 1997; Ries 1997.

14. For example, Davis-Floyd's (1992) analysis of childbirth in the United States argued that medicalization is accomplished through rituals that symbolically convey the superiority of science and technology over nature, which is associated with women and their unpredictable bodies. Davis-Floyd saw biomedical discourses on childbirth enjoying a wide degree of hegemony, for few women with the means of choosing alternative approaches to birth do so. Martin (1987) found differences in working-class and middle-class women's adherence to scientific explanations about their bodies and reproductive processes. She suggested that middle-class women, with more to gain from the acceptance of scientific paradigms, were more likely to invest in them despite their negative implications about the female body. Fraser (1995, 1998) showed how the historical exclusion of African American women from hospital births during segregation paved the way for their later acceptance of the kind of medicalization afforded white middle-class women, a process Fraser depicts as less a matter of "domination" than an ironic sort of victory. See also Ginsburg (1989); Ginsburg and Rapp (1995); Haggis (1998); Inhorn (1994); Kahn (2000); Lock and Kaufert (1998); Ragone (1994); Ram and Jolly (1998); Rapp (1999).

15. It is important to distinguish "the state" as an analytical concept from "our system" as a locally recognized and widely deployed idiom by which state power was made meaningful and experienced. The notion of "our system" appears to refer more specifically to the Soviet bureaucracy than to the state as a whole, because while the bureaucratic face of the socialist system was widely delegitimized and its power seen as immoral, and while it was labeled "our system," I do not assume that people critical of bureaucratic power also completely rejected the state's and socialism. Bureaucratic constraints and bureaucratized forms of interpersonal engagement were one dimension of what people knew of the state, one way in which the state's power and authority became expressed and performed. People who lamented the capricious and unjust actions of "our system" may still have favored, consented to, or supported the larger regime of the Soviet Union, for example.

16. In their comments on this burden, physicians also contributed to the discursive construction of the nation's "dying out."

17. For details on social welfare benefits intended to promote and fertility and family life, see Desfosses (1981); Jones and Grupp (1987: 275); Zakharov (1999); Zakharov and Ivanova (1996).

1. PROMOTING DEMOCRACY THROUGH MORAL CORRECTION

1. This and all other names used in this book are pseudonyms.

2. The Healthy Cities Project official I worked with at WHO in Copenhagen objected to my calling the delegation that worked in St. Petersburg "WHO," inasmuch as these consultants were not funded by the international agency and were not employees of it. I have thus used terms such as "WHO affiliates" or "WHO consultants" in this book. However, their affiliation with the agency, and WHO's technical sponsorship of their project, made the boundary between who and what is and is not WHO fuzzy. Moreover,

the intricacies of global relationships between consultants and agency were unfamiliar to St. Petersburg health providers. In their eyes, the delegation members were WHO representatives.

3. WHO consultants estimated the city's maternal mortality to be as high as 70 per 100,000 live births, in contrast to rates of 6–7 per 100,000 in Western Europe.

4. A WHO report issued following the 1992 Consensus Conference found the following causes of maternal mortality that year: 28% associated with induced abortion outside the official health care system; 26% associated with caesarean section; 25% occurred in the postpartum period with hemorrhage the most frequent complication (WHO 1993b: 3).

5. Almost immediately after the declaration for primary health care was signed by representatives from around the globe, its proponents found themselves having to defend the need to improve general social welfare and reduce economic disparities to improve the health of the poor. In 1979, the idea of "selective primary health care" was proposed as a means of delivering cost-effective interventions to treat the most prevalent diseases (Walsh and Warren 1979). Opponents retorted that such an approach negated the entire concept of primary care set forth in Alma Ata and served largely to uphold the status quo without attending to any significant redistribution of resources (Rifkin and Walt 1986: 560). A vociferous debate developed between those seeking to preserve the more radical implications of primary health care, with its commitment to long-term socioeconomic investments, and those advocating a "realistic" use of medical interventions for rapid results. For other discussions and critiques of the rhetorics and realization of international health development projects, see Donahue 1989; Green 1989, Justice 1986; Morgan 1993; Pigg 1992; Stone 1986; Taylor and Jolly 1988).

6. One recommendation, to reorganize postnatal care procedures to room mothers and babies together, did aim for a structural reform in health services. It is notable that providers who incorporated these changes described their benefit as reducing their own work load, rather than enhancing women's autonomy and power in the hospital setting, as WHO had encouraged.

7. Accordingly, all names below are pseudonyms. Quotations are based on my field notes taken during the workshops and interviews.

8. Episiotomies are vertical incisions made to open the vaginal canal.

9. Obstetricians in Russia generally perform caesarean sections in pairs.

10. Although I sent WHO consultants a written report following their workshop, with an initial analysis of Russian health providers' perspectives, they never responded.

2. STIMULATING PROVIDERS, INDIVIDUALIZING LABOR

1. The Cuban health care system has been shown to have an extensive, advanced tertiary hospital system in addition to extensive and effective primary care (Chomsky 2000: 333; Feinsilver 1993).

2. *Feldshers* are best described as physicians' assistants. Since the 1970s, they have been key to the provision of health care in rural areas.

3. As women were recruited en masse into the paid work force in the years following the Revolution, their activities as workers and mothers were studied and interpreted through metaphors of "production." Hyer (1996) provides fascinating insights into the ways a language of economics became a tool through which Soviet physicians in the 1920s conducted surveillance of women's reproductive and productive capacities. Fertility rates became measures for "labor" productivity, while the quality of labor participation became charted at the site of women's pelvises and menses (1996: 114).

4. This argument is positioned against so-called convergence theorists (such as Ivan Illich 1976), whose critiques assume that the managerial/ technocratic class controls political and economic institutions in all contemporary societies.

5. There were also separate children's outpatient clinics, so no integration of gynecology and pediatrics occurred.

6. The residence registration, or *propiska,* was a central form of Soviet and post-Soviet government surveillance over the population, serving as a means of controlling people and determining their legal rights. Due to the dire housing shortages and the bureaucratic difficulties of attaining and changing residence registrations, people often lived in places other that where they are officially registered. As a result, to attain free health care, it was often necessary to travel long distances back to the neighborhood where they are registered. Several chief doctors of women's clinics told me that they do not check the *propiska* of pregnant women in need of prenatal care, asserting, "We never turn away a pregnant woman" (as opposed to women seeking abortions). Most women, however, were not aware that physicians followed this informal procedure.

7. Also ignored is the role of key U.S.-based development consultants, several of whom have been indicted for fraud in connection with their practices of implementing privatization programs (Cambanis 2002).

8. See Alekseev, Batina, and Abushkin (2002) for an experiment in compensating surgeons according to volume and difficulty of care in Cheliabinsk; see Zel'kovich (1996) for attempts in Kemerovo and Samara oblasts to conceptualize criteria based on "final outcomes" of care.

3. INDIVIDUALIZING DISCIPLINES OF SEX EDUCATION

1. Maternal mortality was 50.2 in 1997, approximately 7 times the rate in the U.S. (Notzon et al. 1999: iv). There were 2,016 abortions for every 1,000 live births in 1997 (Popov and David 1999: 233). The rate of syphilis in 1997, for example, was 277.6 per 100,000, representing an increase of 64.5 times over the 1989 rate of 4.2 (Tichonova et al. 1997; Vishnevskii 2000: 85–86). Gonorrhea and chlamydia were also proliferating. And although few Russians in the mid 1990s acknowledged that HIV posed a serious threat for their country, they received constant warnings from global experts that an explosion of the virus must not be discounted.

2. In 1987, the official rate of abortion in the Soviet Union (a rate that did not take into account substantial numbers of illegal and unregistered abortions) was estimated at 111.9 per 1000 women aged 15–44.

3. This particular set of associations between physical and moral qualities represented a new vision promulgated by the Stalin regime. Traditional notions of the Russian village defined physical dirt as a sign of belonging to the local community and suggested spiritual or moral purity; physical cleanliness had been the cause of moral suspicion (Peterson 1996: 189). The focus on *kul'turnost'* has also stood in contradiction to a long-standing Russian oral folklore tradition of obscene jokes and limericks (*chastushki*), and a rich language of obscenities (*mat'*)—which was often used as a form of oppositional expression under the Soviet regime.

4. Soviet educators were not the first to propose this in Russia. Physicians and educators at the turn of the twentieth century urged sexual restraint as necessary for responsible citizens and an effectively run society (Engelstein 1992b: 225, 245; Field 1996).

5. Attwood argues that the project of sex-role socialization predated the announcement of a demographic crisis, but provided an impetus and justification for pedagogues to propagate their views on the essential, inevitable quality of sex differences in personality

and raise their own status as specialists with important knowledge (1990: 8). While sex-role socialization should not be identified as the same as "sex education," it was practically the only formal genre in which issues remotely related to sexuality ("family life") were conveyed until the mid 1990s. Of course, sexuality and sex per se were not mentioned in these classes. In a later article, Attwood describes sex-role socialization as a "propaganda campaign" (1996: 256). Though a justifiable characterization, it arguably closes inquiry into the ways this campaign may have been creatively implemented by different educators, or even appropriated as an opportunity to address issues connected to "personal hygiene" and "family life" that were not explicitly dictated by the state.

6. In another study (Kon and Riordan 1993: 40), Kon, provides data from a public opinion poll about the desirability of introducing sex education classes in schools. When the question stated that classes would begin at the age of 11 or 12, 61% of women and 58% of men responded favorably to the idea. Of those who were under 25 years, 80% responded positively, while only 38% of those over 60 did.

7. Their attitude toward this endeavor must be seen in comparison with common attitudes toward public service in health education conducted under the Soviet regime. In that context, physicians were obligated to conduct so-called enlightenment work, a responsibility that physicians widely dreaded because they perceived it as taking them away from medicine and into the more overtly ideological realm of "social work" [*obshchestvennaia rabota*]. With the elimination of Party directives concerning the content of all education, sexual moral education is no longer associated in physicians' minds with "enlightenment work" and is seen by many as an exciting, necessary task.

8. Teen pregnancy rates are difficult to determine because the statistical recording of abortions (in particular those provided in private clinics) is grossly incomplete. For women aged 15–19, the officially calculated abortion rate (which does not include those provided in private clinics) was 69 per 1000 in 1991, and 57 per 1000 in 1995 (Goskomstat 1996: 211). Birth rates for women aged 15–19, however, have risen substantially over the last two decades, though they appeared to be leveling off in the mid 1990s. In 1980, there were 43.7 live births per 1000 women aged 15–19; in 1990, the rate had risen to 55.6 per 1000 in this age group; and by 1995, the rate was 45.6 per 1000 (Zakharov and Ivanova 1996: 363; Goskomstat 1996: 180, 219).

9. For similar contentions in the U.S. context, see Ginsburg (1989) and Sobo (1995).

10. Luker's (1984) study of activists in the American abortion debate found that anti-abortion advocates rejected birth control because of the separation it constructs between sexuality and parenthood. They articulated explicit opposition to the notion of preventing and planning pregnancies because such activities implied that sexuality could be geared toward other ends, such as pleasure alone. This concept of sex was interpreted as an attack on the traditional family structure and women's primary role as mother (1984: 163–64). Russian sex educators, in contrast, were not *consciously* opposed to the use of contraception; the teen center provided teenage girls with free birth control pills and family planning counseling, as well as an unlimited supply of condoms for free to any teenager at the clinic. Yet it seems likely that health providers' belief that urgent efforts were needed to combat sexual dissipation and the breakdown of all moral standards led them to focus on the physical and spiritual dangers of abortion, rather than promote birth control and implicitly condone both sexual activity and the indulgence of sex outside of marriage.

11. While health providers demonstrated great concern with the rapid rise of STIs such as syphilis, it is ironic that AIDS went virtually unmentioned, especially given the fact that syphilis is a harbinger of HIV. This, too, I suggest, was likely a reflection of having relied on their own clinical experiences in shaping their lectures. By the midpoint of 1996, fewer than 200 cases of HIV infection had been reported in St. Petersburg, and approxi-

mately 600 were documented in Moscow (Specter 1997). Given this situation, most gynecologists in St. Petersburg had probably not encountered any patients with HIV. In conversations with me, several physicians explained that they considered it a relatively remote,
"foreign" preoccupation.

12. I owe this wording to Melissa Caldwell, and thank her for her keen insights in the
development of this argument.

4. TAKING RESPONSIBILITY FOR OURSELVES

1. The retention of fluids in pregnant women is a sign of toxemia (pre-eclampsia),
one of the most frequently diagnosed complications in Russian maternity care. I asked
Natalia Borisovna how much a woman is supposed to drink and how much weight she is
supposed to gain in the course of a pregnancy. She explained to me that in a healthy
pregnancy, women gain 10–12 kilos (22–26 lbs.). When a patient is in danger of gaining
excessive weight, obstetricians put her on a strict diet intended to minimize fluid intake.
One liter of fluids a day is then considered the ideal.

2. Russian obstetricians used wooden fetoscopes, placing the narrow end directly on
the woman's stomach, while listening through the wide end.

3. Natalia Borisovna explained that her reluctance was based on the fact that steriliza-
tions were usually performed only on women aged 35 and older.

4. Because most pregnancies were not planned through the explicit use and discon-
tinuation of contraception, women often spent much of the first trimester deciding whether
to keep the pregnancy or terminate it. Only after this decision was made would they begin
prenatal care.

5. *Health,* a popular monthly magazine published in the Soviet era by the Ministry of
Public Health.

5. PERSONAL TIES AND THE AUTHORIZATION
OF MEDICAL POWER

1. Key to these studies on the second economy is an assumption that the pervasive-
ness of informal practices reflected the delegitimation of the Soviet regime: to the extent
that ordinary people needed to resort to deceit and subterfuge to fulfill their daily needs,
they ceased believing in the state's ideology of the superiority of the socialist system (Kligman 1998; Verdery 1996). Informal activities that directly disobeyed or indirectly bypassed the law reflected a concern with personal values and interests, as opposed to state or
collective needs. Such practices undermined collectivist principles, chipped away at the
authority of the system, fatally weakened the state, and ultimately lead to the implosion of
the socialist system from within (Verdery 1996). This analysis offered important alternatives to totalitarian models of a strong Soviet state, but it is now becoming clear that
participants in informal practices did not necessarily consider themselves to be "resisting"
official ideology or equate their strategies with a compromise of belief in the Soviet system
(Ledeneva 1998; Yurchak 1997, 2003). Ethnographic analysis can reveal how informal
practices as strategies worked in specific social arenas. The continuing presence of informal
relations in the aftermath of Soviet society also raises the question: if informal and unofficial strategies often expressed dissatisfaction with the Soviet regime, how do we understand their persistence and reconfiguration under market democracy?

2. I describe this hospital's conditions as "socialist" in the mid 1990s because its
budget was entirely funded through public resources and no user fees had been established.

3. The maternity hospital system was organized so that patients could choose to give
birth at any hospital in the city if they arrived with their own transportation. If they came

by ambulance, as many needed to, they would be taken to whatever hospital was "on duty" in their neighborhood. Many women, moreover, preferred to be in the hospital before labor began, in part because the bridges over the Neva River in St. Petersburg detach every evening at 2 A.M., and travel is impossible until they close again at 6 A.M. If your preferred hospital was on the other side of a bridge from your home, and you were not already admitted when labor began, you would end up going somewhere else.

4. Moreover, as Natalia Borisovna and Nina Petrovna revealed in their discussion back in their office, the timing of the exchange also had significance. Offered *before* a woman gives birth, a box of chocolates appeared closer to a bribe; given afterward, it was unmistakably a gift of thanks.

5. The idea that women needed babies to create and cement relationships was applied to single women, too. Doctors and women alike told me that women who do not get married should have a baby anyway, to create a family for themselves. Doctors explained this to me when they described single women who "were giving birth for themselves" [*dlia sebia rozhaiut*]. One physician in her early fifties told me her plans for her 27-year-old single daughter: "I told Sveta, if you don't get married by the time you're 30, we'll have a baby. It's the worst thing to be alone."

6. This was a sign of an infection that could be contagious, which prohibited her staying in the hospital.

6. PRIVATIZING MEDICALIZATION

1. At the time of the interview, I had no reason to doubt the veracity of this price. Yet Oksana, a women interviewed for this project, told me that she paid $200 for an official paid birth at No. 18 in 1994, which suggests that the prices quoted me may not have been standardized for all patients.

2. Maternity hospital No. 6, which had no paid services earlier in the decade, stated that they still provided only free care; but a doctor I met corrected this impression, telling us that her acquaintance worked there and said that for $400—paid unofficially—a woman could choose her doctor ahead of time and then be housed in a postpartum room with only one other patient.

3. St. Petersburg Maternity Hospital, *Family Births.* Retrieved from www.rody.spb.ru/roddom/rody_home.html, accessed 17 August 2001, pp. 1–13.

4. Ibid.

5. Ibid., 5.

6. For similar processes occurring in rural China, see Farquhar 1996.

CONCLUSION

1. In response to this situation, Russian health policy observers associated with the IMF advised revisions in the scope of compulsory health insurance guarantees to be more in line with budgetary realities, rather than to restructure the budget to maintain these minimal services (Dmitriev et al. 2000: 1).

2. In early elaborations of this argument during the 1980s, Antonov argued against fellow demographers who emphasized the need to improve families' material conditions, such as housing, as the central means for increasing the birth rate. It was not economic need that prevented families from bearing two or three children, he insisted, for social sectors with the worst material conditions have, on average, larger numbers of children than the more highly educated, professional elites (Antonov and Medkov 1987).

3. The pejorative associations with feminism are hardly unique to Russia, of course. On the backlash against feminism in the U.S., see Faludi (1992). Even in Western Europe,

where social welfare policies advantageous to women's issues such as childcare have been strongly promoted, activists eschew discourses claiming them as "feminist" issues, preferring seemingly more inclusive labels as "universalism" (Hautanen 2003; Natkin 2003).

4. I owe this wording to Linda Gordon, who made a similar comment at the 2003 Bruno Kreisky Archive Conference on the "Gender of Politics," Vienna, Austria.

5. Of course, there are other reasons that feminism has been marginal in former socialist societies, foremost of which is the fact that the socialist project itself appropriated feminist language of women's "emancipation" and "equality" while mobilizing women's labor and reproductive potentials for its own purposes. A result of this experience was that feminist language became widely discredited, and little consciousness of gender inequality developed.

6. I do not mean to suggest that concerns with health and safety have not been central to liberal feminist arguments in the West. Rather, I feel that it may be necessary to take conscious, strategic steps to counter negative associations stemming from feminists' connections with liberal individualism, by highlighting these kinds of welfare issues more than they have been to date.

7. On the ways this dichotomy plays out in demographic debates, see Rivkin-Fish 2003.

8. I realize that one danger in relying on consumer groups is the fact that not all health service users have the same interests, and women from marginalized groups (such as the poor, refugees, and ethnic minorities) may have their needs excluded from the agendas of such groups.

WORKS CITED

Abbott, Andrew D. 1988. *The System of Professions: An Essay on the Division of Expert Labor.* Chicago: University of Chicago Press.

Abramson, David. 1999. "A Critical Look at NGOs and Civil Society as Means to an End in Uzbekistan." *Human Organization* 58(3): 240–250.

Alekseev, N. A., N. P. Batina, and I. A. Abushkin. 2002. "Ob oplate truda vrachei khirurgicheskikh spetsial'nostei." *Problemy sotsial'noi gigieny, zdravookhraneniia i istorii meditsiny* 1: 37–39.

Alma Ata. 1978. *Primary Health Care.* Health for All Series, no. 1. Geneva: World Health Organization.

Antonov, A. I. 1980. *Sotsiologiia rozhdaemosti: Teoreticheskie i metodologicheskie problemy.* Moscow: Statistika.

———. 1982. *Sem'ia i deti.* Moscow: Izdatel'stvo Moskovskogo Universiteta.

———. 1986. *Demograficheskoe povedenie i vozmozhnosti sotsial'nogo vozdeistviia na nego v usloviiakh sotsializma: po materialam mezhdunarodnoi nauchno-prakticheskoi konferentsii v Vilniuse, 1985 g.* Moscow: Akademiia nauk SSSR Institut sotsio-logicheskikh issledovanii.

———. 1995. "Sem'ia kak institut sredi drugikh sotsial'nykh institutov." In *Sem'ia na poroge tret'ego tysiacheletiia,* ed. A. I. Antonov and V. V. Negodin, 182–198. Moscow: Institut sotsiologii Rossiiskoi Akademii Nauk, Tsentr obshchechelovecheskikh tsennostei.

Antonov, A. I., and V. M. Medkov. 1987. *Vtoroi rebenok.* Moscow: Mysl'.

Antonov, A. I., and S. A. Sorokin. 2002. *Sud'ba sem'i v Rossii XXI veka.* Moscow: Graal'.

Ashwin, Sarah. 1999. "Redefining the Collective: Russian Mineworkers in Transition." In *Uncertain Transition: Ethnographies of Change in the Postsocialist World,* ed. M. Burawoy and K. Verdery. Lanham, Md.: Rowman and Littlefield.

Ashwin, Sarah, ed. 2000. *Gender, State and Society in Soviet and Post-Soviet Russia.* London: Routledge.

Attwood, Lynne. 1990. *The New Soviet Man and Woman: Sex Role Socialization in the USSR.* London: Macmillan in association with the Centre for Russian and East European Studies, University of Birmingham.

———. 1996. "The Post-Soviet Woman in the Move to the Market: A Return to Domesticity and Dependence?" In *Women in Russia and Ukraine,* ed. R.J. Marsh, 255–266. New York: Cambridge University Press.

Babasyan, Natalya. 1995. "Freedom or 'Life': Secular and Russian Orthodox Organiza-tions Unite in a Struggle against Reproductive Freedom for Women." *Izvestiia,* 26 February 1999, 5. Reprinted in *Current Digest of the Post-Soviet Press* (hereafter *CDPSP*) 51(12): 4, 6.

Baidan, Natalya. 1999. "You Have to Save Up to Have a Baby." *Vremia MN,* 24 August 1999, 3. Reprinted in *CDPSP* 51(36): 16–17.

Ballaeva, E. A. 1998. *Gendernaia ekspertiza zakonodatel'stva RF: Reproduktivnye prava zhenshchin v Rossii.* Moscow: MTSGI (Moscow Center for Gender Studies).

Barker, Adele Marie, ed. 1999. *Consuming Russia: Popular Culture, Sex, and Society since Gorbachev.* Durham, N.C.: Duke University Press.

Barr, Donald A., and Mark Field. 1996. "The Current State of Health Care in the Former Soviet Union: Implication for Health Care Policy and Reform." *American Journal of Public Health* 86(3): 307–312.

Bassom, Ann. 1999. "The Russian Press: Coverage of Women's Health." In *Medical Issues and Health Care Reform in Russia,* ed. V. L. Hesli and M. H. Mills, 233–263. Lewiston, N.Y.: Edwin Mellen Press.

Bateneva, Tat'iana. 1997. "Na sobach'em urovne." *Izvestiia,* 1 April, p. 5.

———. 1998. "Nevezhestvo pod vidom bioetiki." *Izvestiia,* 13 Oct., pp. 1, 7.

Berdahl, Daphne, Matti Bunzl, and Martha Lampland, eds. 2000. *Altering States: Ethnographies of Transition in Eastern Europe and the Former Soviet Union.* Ann Arbor: University of Michigan Press.

Bourdieu, Pierre 1977. *Outline of a Theory of Practice.* New York: Cambridge University Press.

———. 1990. *The Logic of Practice.* Stanford, Calif.: Stanford University Press.

———. 1994. "Rethinking the State: Genesis and Structure of the Bureaucratic Field." *Sociological Theory* 12(1): 1–18.

Boym, Svetlana. 1994. *Common Places: Mythologies of Everyday Life in Russia.* Cambridge, Mass.: Harvard University Press.

Bridger, Sue, Rebecca Kay, and Kathryn Pinnick. 1996. *No More Heroines? Russia, Women, and the Market.* New York: Routledge.

Briggs, Charles. 1986. *Learning How to Ask.* Cambridge: Cambridge University Press.

Brown, Julie V., and Nina L. Rusinova. 1997. "Russian Medical Care in the 1990s: A User's Perspective." *Social Science and Medicine* 45(8): 1265–1276.

———. 2000. "Negotiating the Post-Soviet Medical Marketplace: Growing Gaps in the Safety Net." In *Russia's Torn Safety Nets,* ed. M. Field and J. Twigg, 65–82. New York: St. Martin's Press.

Bourdieu, Pierre. 1977. *Outline of a Theory of Practice.* New York: Cambridge University Press.

———. 1994. "Rethinking the State: Genesis and Structure of the Bureaucratic Field." *Sociological Theory* 12(1): 1-18.

Buchowski, Michał. 2001. *Rethinking Transformation: An Anthropological Perspective on Postsocialism.* Poznan: Wydawnictwo Humaniora.

Bunton, Robin, and Gordon Macdonald, eds. 1992. *Health Promotion: Disciplines and Diversity.* New York: Routledge.

Burawoy, Michael, Pavel Krotov, and Tatyana Lytkina. 2000. "Involution and Destitution in Capitalist Russia." *Ethnography* 1(1): 43–65.

Burawoy, Michael, and Katherine Verdery, eds. 1999. *Uncertain Transition: Ethnographies of Change in the Postsocialist World.* Lanham, Md.: Rowman and Littlefield.

Caldwell, Melissa L. 2004. *Not by Bread Alone: Social Support in the New Russia.* Berkeley: University of California Press.

Cambanis, Thanassis. 2002. "Prosecutors Argue Harvard Owes US at Least $34m in Russia Case." *Boston Globe,* 18 December. Reprinted on Johnson's Russia List, no. 6606. 18 December 2002, no. 1.

Caplan, Ronald L., Donald W. Light, and Norman Daniels. 1999. "Benchmarks of Fairness: A Moral Framework for Assessing Equity." *International Journal of Health Services* 29(4): 853–869.

Chesanova, T. 1994. "Bolet' v Peterburge opasno dlia zhizni." *Chas Pik* 26 (October): 1.

Chomsky, Aviva. 2000. "'The Threat of a Good Example': Health and Revolution in Cuba." In *Dying for Growth: Global Inequality and the Health of the Poor,* ed. J. Yong Kim, J. Millen, A. Irwin, and J. Gershman, 331–358. Monroe, Maine: Common Courage Press.

Cohen, Stephen. 2000. *Failed Crusade: America and the Tragedy of Post-Communist Russia.* New York: W.W. Norton.

Comaroff, Jean. 1982. "Medicine: Symbol and Ideology." In *The Problem of Medical Knowledge,* ed. P. Wright and A. Treacher, 49–68. Edinburgh: Edinburgh University Press.

———. 1985. *Body of Power, Spirit of Resistance: The Culture and History of a South African People.* Chicago: University of Chicago Press.

Curtis, Sarah, N. Petukhova, and A. Taket. 1995. "Health Care Reforms in Russia: The Example of St. Petersburg." *Social Science and Medicine* 40(6): 755–765.

Curtis, Sarah, Natasha Petukhova, Galina Sezonova, and Nadia Netsenko. 1997. "Caught in the 'Traps of Managed Competition'? Examples of Russian Health Care Reforms from St. Petersburg and the Leningrad Region." *International Journal of Health Services* 27(4): 661–686.

Das, Veena, et al., eds. 2001. *Remaking a World: Violence, Social Suffering, and Recovery.* Berkeley: University of California Press.

Davis-Floyd, Robbie. 1992. *Birth as an American Rite of Passage.* Berkeley: Berkeley University Press.

de George, R. T. 1969. *Soviet Ethics and Morality.* Ann Arbor: University of Michigan Press.

Delovoi Peterburg 2000. "Kak delat' detei, Peterburg znaet. No ne mozhet." June 22, pp. 8–9.

Derzhavina, Olga. 1998. "Russia Has 100 Years to Live: The Country Is Experiencing an Unprecedented Crisis." *Segodnia,* December 7, pp. 1–2. Reprinted in *CDPSP* 50(49): 16.

Desfosses, Helen. 1976. "Demography, Ideology, and Politics in the USSR." *Soviet Studies* 28(2): 244–256.

———. 1981. "Pro-Natalism in Soviet Law and Propaganda." In *Soviet Population Policy: Conflicts and Constraints,* ed. H. Desfosses. New York: Pergamon Press.

Dmitriev, Mikhail, Yelena Potapchik, Olga Solovieva, and Sergei Shishkin. 2000. "Economic Problems of Health Services Reform in Russia." Retrieved from www.imf.org/external/pubs/ft/seminar/2000/pdf/dmitriev2.pdf, accessed 19 April 2002.

Donahue, John M. 1989. "International Organizations, Health Services, and Nation Building in Nicaragua." *Medical Anthropology Quarterly* 3(3): 258–269.

Dunham, Vera S. 1990 [1976]. *In Stalin's Time: Middleclass Values in Soviet Fiction.* New York: Cambridge University Press.

Dunn, Elizabeth. 1999. "Slick Salesmen and Simple People: Negotiated Capitalism in a Privatized Polish Firm." In *Uncertain Transition: Ethnographies of Change in the Postsocialist World,* ed. M. Burawoy and K. Verdery. Lanham, Md.: Rowman and Littlefield.

———. 2004. *Privatizing Poland: Baby Food, Big Business, and the Remaking of the Polish Working Class.* Ithaca, N.Y.: Cornell University Press.

Eberstadt, Nicholas. 1999. "Russia: Too Sick to Matter?" *Policy Review* (June–July). Retrieved from www.policyreview.org/jun99/eberstadt_print.html, accessed 21 December 2001.

234 | Works Cited

Eckstein, Harry. 1960. *Pressure Group Politics: The Case of the British Medical Association.* Stanford, Calif.: Stanford University Press.

Engelstein, Laura. 1992a. "There Is Sex in Russia—and Always Was: Some Recent Contributions to Russian Erotica." *Slavic Review* 51(4): 786–790.

———. 1992b. *The Keys to Happiness: Sex and the Search for Modernity in Fin-de-siècle Russia.* Ithaca, N.Y.: Cornell University Press.

Escobar, Arturo. 1995. *Encountering Development: The Making and Unmaking of the Third World.* Princeton, N.J.: Princeton University Press.

Faludi, Susan. 1992. *Backlash: The Undeclared War against American Women.* New York: Anchor Books.

Farmer, Paul. 1992. *AIDS and Accusation: Haiti and the Geography of Blame.* Berkeley: University of California Press.

———. 1999. *Infections and Inequalities: The Modern Plagues.* Berkeley: University of California Press.

Farquhar, Judith. 1996. "Market Magic: Getting Rich and Getting Personal in Medicine after Mao." *American Ethnologist* 23(2): 239-257.

Feinsilver, Julie Margot. 1993. *Healing the Masses: Cuban Health Politics at Home and Abroad.* Berkeley: University of California Press.

Ferguson, James. 1994. *The Anti-Politics Machine: "Development," Depoliticization, and Bureaucratic Power in Lesotho.* Minneapolis: University of Minnesota Press.

Field, Deborah Ann. 1996. "Communist Morality and Meanings of Private Life in Post-Stalinist Russia, 1953–1964." Ph.D. dissertation, University of Michigan.

Field, Mark. 1957. *Doctor and Patient in Russia.* Cambridge, Mass.: Harvard University Press.

———. 1991. "The Hybrid Profession: Soviet Medicine." In *Professions and the States: Expertise and Autonomy in the Soviet Union and Eastern Europe,* ed. A. Jones, 43–62. Philadelphia: Temple University Press.

———. 1995. "The Health Crisis in the Former Soviet Union: A Report from the 'Post-War' Zone." *Social Science and Medicine* 41(11): 1469–1478.

Field, Mark, David M. Kotz, and Gene Bukhman. 2000. "Neoliberal Economic Policy, 'State Desertion,' and the Russian Health Crisis." In *Dying for Growth: Global Inequality and the Health of the Poor,* ed. J. Y. Kim, J. V. Millen, A. Irwin, and J. Gershman, 155–173. Monroe, Maine: Common Courage Press.

Field, Mark, and Judyth Twigg. 2000. "Introduction." In *Russia's Torn Safety Nets,* ed. M. Field and J. Twigg, 1–10. New York: St. Martin's Press.

Foucault, Michel. 1973. *Madness and Civilization: A History of Insanity in the Age of Reason.* New York: Vintage Books.

———. 1980. *The History of Sexuality.* New York: Pantheon Books.

———. 1988. "Technologies of the Self." In *Technologies of the Self: A Seminar with Michel Foucault,* ed. L. H. Martin et al., 16–49. Amherst: University of Massachusetts Press.

Fraser, Gertrude J. 1995. "Modern Bodies, Modern Minds: Midwifery and Reproductive Change in an African American Community." In *Conceiving the New World Order: The Global Politics of Reproduction,* ed. F. Ginsburg and R. Rapp, 42–58. Berkeley: University of California Press.

———. 1998. *African American Midwifery in the South: Dialogues of Birth, Race, and Memory.* Cambridge, Mass.: Harvard University Press.

Freidson, Eliot. 1986 [1970]. *Profession of Medicine: A Study of the Sociology of Applied Knowledge.* New York: Harper and Row.

———. 1994. *Professionalism Reborn: Theory, Prophecy, and Policy.* Cambridge: Polity Press.

Funk, Nanette. 1993. "Introduction" in *Gender Politics and Post-Communism: Reflections from Eastern Europe and the Former Soviet Union*, ed. Nanette Funk and Magda Mueller, 1–14. New York: Routledge.

Funk, Nanette, and Magda Mueller, eds. 1993. *Gender Politics and Postcommunism: Reflections from Eastern Europe and the Former Soviet Union.* New York: Routledge.

Gal, Susan. 1994. "Gender in the Post-Socialist Transition: The Abortion Debate in Hungary." *East European Politics and Societies* 8(2): 256–286.

———. 1997. "Feminism and Civil Society." In *Transitions, Environments, Translations: Feminisms in International Politics,* ed. J. Scott, C. Kaplan, and D. Keates, 30–45. New York: Routledge.

Gal, Susan, and Gail Kligman. 2000a. *The Politics of Gender after Socialism.* Princeton, N.J.: Princeton University Press.

———. 2000b. *Reproducing Gender: Politics, Publics, and Everyday Life after Socialism.* Princeton, N.J.: Princeton University Press.

Ginsburg, Faye. 1989. *Contested Lives: The Abortion Debate in an American Community.* Berkeley: University of California Press.

Ginsburg, Faye, and Rayna Rapp. 1995. "Introduction: Conceiving the New World Order." In *Conceiving the New World Order: The Global Politics of Reproduction,* ed. F. Ginsburg and R. Rapp, 1–18. Berkeley: University of California Press.

Goldman, Wendy Z. 1993. *Women, the State, and Revolution: Soviet Family Policy and Social Life, 1917–1936.* New York: Cambridge University Press.

Golukhov, G. N., A. Iu. Shilenko, and Iu. V. Shilenko. 1996. "Razvitie negosudarstven-nogo sektora zdravookhraneniia v perekhodnoi ekonomike." *Problemy sotsial'noi gigieny, zdravookhraneniia i istorii meditsiny* 6: 25–31.

Good, Byron. 1994. *Medicine, Rationality, and Experience: An Anthropological Perspective.* Cambridge, N.Y.: Cambridge University Press.

Goscilo, Helena. 1993. "Domostroika or Perestroika? The Construction of Womanhood in Soviet Culture under Glasnost." In *Late Soviet Culture: From Perestroika to Novostroika,* ed. T. Lahusen with G. Kuperman, 233–255. Durham, N.C.: Duke University Press.

Goscilo, Helena, and Beth Holmgren, eds. 1996. *Russia • Women • Culture.* Bloomington: Indiana University Press.

Goskomstat (Gosudarstvennyi komitet Rossiiskoi Federatsii po statistike). 1996. *Demograficheskii ezhegodnik Rossii* (The Demographic Yearbook of Russia). Moscow: Goskomstat.

Green, Linda Buckley. 1989. "Consensus and Coercion: Primary Health Care and the Guatemalan State." *Medical Anthropology Quarterly* 3(3): 246–257.

Gridasova, I. 1994. "Khochesh' lechit'sia-ishchi sponsora." *Sankt-Peterburgskie vedomosti* 16 (October): 1.

Grigor'ev, F. G. 1995. "Uchrezhdeniia zdravookhraneniia v usloviiakh rynka." *Problemy sotsial'noi gigieny, zdravookhraneniia i istorii meditsiny* 2: 49–51.

Gupta, Akhil. 1995. "Blurred Boundaries: The Discourse of Corruption, the Culture of Politics, and the Imagined State." *American Ethnologist* 22(2): 375–402.

Haggis, Jane. 1998. "'Good Wives and Mothers' or 'Dedicated Workers'? Contradictions of Domesticity in the 'Mission of Sisterhood,' Travancore, South India." In *Maternities and Modernities: Colonial and Postcolonial Experiences in Asia and the Pacific,* ed. K. Ram and M. Jolly, 81–113. Cambridge: Cambridge University Press.

Hann, Chris, and Elizabeth Dunn, eds. 1996. *Civil Society: Challenging Western Models.* New York: Routledge.

Hautanen, Teija. 2003. "Every Child's Right to Public Daycare in Finland." Paper Presented at the conference "The Gender of Politics: The Example of Reproduction

Politics in Austria, Finland, Portugal, Romania, Russia, and the US Bruno Kreisky Archive, Vienna, Austria," 14 March 2003.

Havelkova, Hana. 1993. "A Few Prefeminist Thoughts." In *Gender Politics and Post-Communism: Reflections from Eastern Europe and the Former Soviet Union,* 62–73. New York: Routledge.

Hemment, Julie. 2000. "Gender, NGOs and the Third Sector in Russia: An Ethnography of Post-Socialist Civil Society." Ph.D. dissertation, Cornell University.

———. 2004a. "Strategizing Development: Translations, Appropriations, Responsibilities." In *Post-Soviet Women Encountering Transition: Nation Building, Economic Survival, and Civic Activism,* ed. K. Kuehnast and C. Nechemias, 313–334. Baltimore and Washington, D.C.: Johns Hopkins University Press and Woodrow Wilson International Center for Scholars Press.

———. 2004b. "Global Civil Society and the Local Costs of Belonging: Defining Violence against Women in Russia." *Signs: Journal of Women in Culture and Society* 29(3): 815–840.

Herzfeld, Michael. 1993. *The Social Production of Indifference: Exploring the Symbolic Roots of Western Bureaucracy.* Chicago: University of Chicago Press.

Human Life International. 2001. *Culture of Life Being Rebuilt in Russia.* Retrieved from http://www.hli.org/Content/Dynamic/Articles/000/000/000/756biwba.asp, accessed 25 July 2001.

Humphrey, Caroline. 1983. *Karl Marx Collective: Economy, Society, and Religion in a Siberian Collective Farm.* Cambridge: Cambridge University Press.

———. 2002. *The Unmaking of Soviet Life: Everyday Economics after Socialism.* Ithaca, N.Y.: Cornell University Press.

Hyer, Janet. 1996. "Managing the Female Organism: Doctors and the Medicalization of Women's Paid Work in Soviet Russia in the 1920s." In *Women in Russia and Ukraine,* ed. R. J. Marsh. New York: Cambridge University Press.

Illich, Ivan. 1976. *Limits to Medicine: Medical Nemesis: The Expropriation of Health.* London: Marion Boyars.

Inhorn, Marcia. 1994. *Quest for Conception: Gender, Infertility, and Egyptian Medical Traditions.* Philadelphia: University of Pennsylvania Press.

Johnson, Janet. 2004. "Sisterhood vs. the 'Moral' Russian State: The Post-Communist Politics of Rape." In *Post-Soviet Women Encountering Transition: Nation Building, Economic Survival, and Civic Activism,* ed. K. Kuehnast and C. Nechemias. Baltimore and Washington, D.C.: Johns Hopkins University Press and Woodrow Wilson International Center for Scholars Press.

Jones, Anthony, and Elliot A. Krause. 1991. "Professions, the State, and the Reconstruction of Socialist Societies." In *Professions and the State: Expertise and Autonomy in the Soviet Union and Eastern Europe,* ed. A. Jones, 233–254. Philadelphia: Temple University Press.

Jones, Ellen, and Fred W. Grupp. 1987. *Modernization, Value Change and Fertility in the Soviet Union.* Cambridge: Cambridge University Press.

Justice, Judith. 1986. *Policies, Plans and People: Culture and Health Development in Nepal.* Berkeley: University of California Press.

Kahn, Susan Martha. 2000. *Reproducing Jews: A Cultural Account of Assisted Conception in Israel.* Durham, N.C.: Duke University Press.

Kay, Rebecca. 2000a. "Zhenshchina-Mat'. Russian Women's Responses to Motherhood: Natural Destiny, National Duty or Personal Choice?" Paper presented to Panel XI-10, "Motherhood, Nationalism and the Reproduction of Inequality II," VI ICCEESS World Congress, Tampere, Finland.

―――. 2000b. *Russian Women and Their Organizations: Gender, Discrimination and Grassroots Women's Organizations, 1991–96.* London: Palgrave Macmillan.

Kennedy, Michael. 2002. *Cultural Formations of Postcommunism: Emancipation, Transition, Nation, and War.* Minneapolis: University of Minnesota Press.

Kharkhordin, Oleg. 1999. *The Collective and the Individual in Russia: A Study of Practices.* Berkeley: University of California Press.

Khipkovoi, A. G., B. Z. Vul'fov, and I. V. Grebennikov, eds. 1982. *Podrostok.* Moscow: Pedagogika.

Khorev, Boris. 1995. "Rynok: podi pri nem rodi. . . ." *Pravda,* March 30, pp. 1–2.

―――. 1997. "V chem ostrota demograficheskoi problemy v Rossii?" *Rossiia i Mir (Informatsionnyi ekspress biulleten' dlia deputatov Gosudarstvennoi Dumy).* Communist Party of the Russian Federation, June, pp. 1–45.

Kleinman, Arthur. 1973. "Medicine's Symbolic Reality: On the Central Problem in the Philosophy of Medicine." *Inquiry* 16: 206–213.

―――. 1980. *Patients and Healers in the Context of Culture: An Exploration of the Borderland between Anthropology, Medicine, and Psychiatry.* Berkeley: University of California Press.

―――. 1988. *The Illness Narratives: Suffering, Healing and the Human Condition.* New York: Basic Books.

―――. 1995. *Writing at the Margin: Discourse between Anthropology and Medicine.* Berkeley: University of California Press.

Kleinman, Arthur, Veena Das, and Margaret Lock, eds. 1997. *Social Suffering.* Berkeley: University of California Press.

Kligman, Gail. 1998. *The Politics of Duplicity: Controlling Reproduction in Ceausescu's Romania.* Berkeley: University of California Press.

Kon, Igor Semenovich. 1995. *The Sexual Revolution in Russia: From the Age of Czars to Today.* New York: Free Press.

Kon, Igor Semenovich, and James Riordan, eds. 1993. *Sex and Russian Society.* London: Pluto Press.

Krause, Elliot A. 1991. "Professions and the State in the Soviet Union and Eastern Europe." In *Professions and the State: Expertise and Autonomy in the Soviet Union and Eastern Europe,* ed. A. Jones, 3–42. Philadelphia: Temple University Press.

Krueger, Anne. 2002. "Growth and Reform in Russia." Address given to the International Monetary Fund, "Conference on Post-Communist Economic Growth," Moscow, March 20. Retrieved from http://www.imf.org/external/np/speeches/2002/032002.htm, accessed 9 April 2002.

Kudrin, V. C., and V. G. Leizerman. 2002. "Otsenka proizvodstvennoi deiatel'nosti i motivatsiia truda v zdravookhranenii." *Problemy sotsial'noi gigieny, zdravookhraneniia i istorii meditsiny* 1: 18–21.

Kvasha, A. Ia. 1981. *Demograficheskaia politika v SSSR.* Moscow: Financy i Statistika.

Lampland, Martha. 2002. "Comments on *The Politics of Gender after Socialism.*" Paper presented at the Council for European Studies Meetings, 15 March.

Lapidus, Gail Warshofsky. 1978. *Women in Soviet Society: Equality, Development, and Social Change.* Berkeley: University of California Press.

Lazarus, Ellen S. 1990. "Falling through the Cracks: Contradictions and Barriers to Care in a Prenatal Clinic." *Medical Anthropology* 12(3): 269–287.

Ledeneva, Alena V. 1998. *Russia's Economy of Favours: Blat, Networking, and Informal Exchange.* Cambridge: Cambridge University Press.

Lemke, Thomas. 2000. "Foucault, Governmentality, and Critique." Paper presented at the "Rethinking Marxism" Conference, University of Massachusetts, Amherst, 21–

24 September. Retrieved from thomaslemkeweb.de/publications-engl.htm on 21 April 2004.

Lemon, Alaina. 2000. *Between Two Fires: Gypsy Performance and Romani Memory from Pushkin to Postsocialism.* Durham, N.C.: Duke University Press.

Light, Donald W. 1995. "*Homo economicus:* Escaping the Traps of Managed Competition." *European Journal of Public Health* 5: 145–154.

———. 2000. "Sociological Perspectives on Competition in Health Care." *Journal of Health Politics, Policy and Law* 25(5): 969–974.

Lindenbraten, A. L., and T. V. Gololobova. 2002. "Uchastie naseleniia v oplate meditsinskoi pomoshchi." *Problemy sotsial'noi gigieny, zdravookhraneniia i istorii meditsiny* 1: 21–24.

Lock, Margaret, and Patricia Kaufert, eds. 1998. *Pragmatic Women and Body Politics.* New York: Cambridge University Press.

Loseva, O. K. 1990. *Polovoe vospitanie detei i podrostkov v sem'e.* Moscow: Ministerstva Zdravookhraneniia SSSR, Filial Gorodskogo Tsentra Zdorovia.

Luker, Kristin. 1984. *Abortion and the Politics of Motherhood.* Berkeley: University of California Press.

Lupton, Deborah. 1995. *The Imperative of Health: Public Health and the Regulated Body.* London: Sage Publications.

Maksimova, T. M., and O. N. Gaenko. 2001. "Meditsinskoe obespechenie naseleniia v usloviiakh sotsial'noi differentsiatsii v obshchestve." *Problemy sotsial'noi gigieny, zdravookhraneniia i istorii meditsiny* 3: 10–14.

Malakhova, Alla. 1999. "'Tsvety zhizni' vianut na glazakh: Pediatry konstatiruiut povsemesnuiu fizicheskuiu i umstvennuiu degredatsiiu russkikh detei." *Novye Izvestiia,* 21 January, 1, 5. Reprinted in the *CDPSP* 51(9): 7–8.

Maleck-Lewy, Eva, and Myra Marx Feree. 2000. "Talking about Women and Wombs: The Discourse of Abortion and Reproductive Rights in the GDR during and after the *Wende.*" In *Reproducing Gender: Politics, Publics and Everyday Life after Socialism,* ed. S. Gal and G. Kligman. Princeton, N.J.: Princeton University Press.

Martin, Emily. 1987. *The Woman in the Body: A Cultural Analysis of Reproduction.* Boston: Beacon Press.

Mead, Margaret. 1954. "The Swaddling Hypothesis: Its Reception." *American Anthropologist* 56: 395–409.

Medvedeva, Irina, and Tat'iana Shishova. 2000. "Demograficheskaia voina protiv Rossii." *Nash Sovremennik,* no. 1. Accessed from http://nashsovr.aihs.net December 22, 2000.

Molodtsova, Viktoria. 1999. "Seks: Razvrashchenie vmesto prosveshcheniia." *Rossiiskaia gazeta,* 9 June, p. 8.

Morgan, Lynn M. 1993. *Community Participation in Health: Primary Health Care in Costa Rica.* New York: Cambridge University Press.

Moscow Center for Gender Studies. 2001. Newsletter. April. MCGS: ISESP/MCGS Russian Academy of Sciences.

Myers, Steven. 2003. "After Decades, Russia Narrows Grounds for Abortions." *New York Times,* 24 August.

Natkin, Ritva. 2001. "A Contradiction between Gender Equality and Protection of Motherhood: Reproduction Policy in Finland." Paper presented at the conference "The Gender of Politics: The Example of Reproduction Politics in Austria, Finland, Portugal, Romania, Russia, and the US," Bruno Kreisky Archive, Vienna, Austria, 14 March 2003.

Navarro, Vincent. 1977. *Social Security and Medicine in the USSR: A Marxist Critique.* Lexington, Mass.: Lexington Books.

Nechemias, Carol. 2000. "Politics in Post-Soviet Russia: Where Are the Women?" *Demokratizatsiia* 8(2): 199–218.

Notzon, F. C., Y. M. Komarov, A. V. Korotkova, S. P. Ermakov, et al. 1999. "Maternal and Child Health Statistics: Russian Federation and United States, Selected Years, 1985–95." Vital Health Statistics, Series 5, International Vital and Health Statistics Report, no. 10.

Ovcharov, V. K., and V. O. Shechepin. 1996. "Neobkhodimost' strukturnykh peremen i ikh mediko-ekonomicheskie tendentsii v zdravookhranenii." *Problemy sotsial'noi gigieny, zdravookhraneniia i istorii meditsiny* 4: 24a–32.

Paley, Julia. 2001. *Marketing Democracy: Power and Social Movements in Post-Dictatorship Chile.* Berkeley: University of California Press.

Perepletchikov, L. 1994. "Podniat' avtoritet professii." *Meditsinskaia gazeta* 18(2): 2.

Pesman, Dale. 2000. *Russia and Soul: An Exploration.* Ithaca, N.Y.: Cornell University Press.

Petersen, Alan, and Robin Bunton, eds. 1997. *Foucault, Health and Medicine.* London: Routledge.

Peterson, Nayda L. 1996. "Dirty Women: Cultural Connotations of Cleanliness in Soviet Russia." In *Russia • Women • Culture,* ed. H. Goscilo and B. Holmgren, 177–208. Bloomington: Indiana University Press.

Petryna, Adriana. 2002. *Life Exposed: Biological Citizenship after Chernobyl.* Princeton, N.J.: Princeton University Press.

Pigg, Stacey Leigh. 1992. "Inventing Social Categories through Place: Social Representations and Development in Nepal." *Comparative Studies in Society and History* 34(3): 491–513.

Pogorelov, Ia. D., and I. E. Chudinova. 1996. "Mediko-sotsial'naia politika kak sostavnaia chast' strategii razvitiia sovremennogo zdravookhraneniia v Rossii." *Problemy sotsial'noi gigieny, zdravookhraneniia i istorii meditsiny* 2: 41–43.

Pokrovskii,V. I., O. P. Shchepin, V. K. Ovcharov, and V. C. Nechaev. 1995. "Osnovnye polozheniia kontseptsii razvitiia zdravookhraneniia Rossii i ego zakonodatel'noe obespechenie." *Problemy sotsial'noi gigieny, zdravookhraneniia I istorii meditsiny* 4: 4–7.

Popov, Andrej A. 1992. "Induced Abortions in the USSR at the End of the 1980's: The Basis for the National Model of Family Planning." Unpublished paper.

Popov, Andrej, and Henry David. 1999. "Russian Federation and USSR Successor States." In *From Abortion to Contraception: A Resource to Public Policies and Reproductive Behavior in Central and Eastern Europe from 1917 to the Present,* ed. Henry P. David, 223–277. Westport, Conn.: Greenwood Press.

Posadskaia, A. I. 1992. "Tendentsii izmeneniia zakonodatel'stva v oblasti sotsial'noi zashchity materinstva." In *Zhenshchiny i sotsial'naia politika: gendernyi aspekt,* ed. Z. A. Khotkina, 79–88. Moscow: Institut sotsial'no-ekonomicheskikh problem narodonaseleniia.

Pravdu.ru. 2003. "Russia Is Given Up for Lost." 29 January. Reprinted in Johnson's Russia List, no. 7040 (30 January 2003).

Public Health Committee of the Mayor's Office of St. Petersburg. 1994. "Reformy zdravookhranenia/The Reform of Medical Health Care" Service [bilingual Russian and English]. St. Petersburg, Russia: Mayor's Office.

Ragone, Helena. 1994. *Surrogate Motherhood: Conception in the Heart.* Boulder: Westview Press.

Ram, Kalpana, and Margaret Jolly, eds. 1998. *Maternities and Modernities: Colonial and Postcolonial Experiences in Asia and the Pacific.* Cambridge: Cambridge University Press.

Rapp, Rayna. 1999. *Testing Women, Testing the Fetus: The Social Impact of Amniocentesis in America.* New York: Routledge.

Remennick, Larissa. 1991. "Epidemiology and Determinants of Induced Abortion in the USSR." *Social Science and Medicine* 33(7): 841–848.

———. 1993. "Patterns of Birth Control." In *Sex and Russian Society,* ed. I. Kon and J. Riordan, 45–63. London: Pluto Press.

Rethman, Petra. 2001. *Tundra Passages: Gender and History in the Russian Far East.* University Park: Pennsylvania State University Press.

Ries, Nancy. 1997. *Russian Talk: Culture and Conversation during Perestroika.* Ithaca, N.Y.: Cornell University Press.

Rifkin, Susan B., and Gil Walt. 1986. "Why Health Improves: Defining the Issues Concerning 'Comprehensive Primary Health Care' and 'Selective Primary Health Care.'" *Social Science and Medicine* 23(6): 559–566.

Rivkin-Fish, Michele. 1994. "Communist Transformations and Abortion Politics: Reflections on Feminist Strategies and 'Choice.'" *Critical Matrix* 8(2): 101–126.

———. 1999. "Sexuality Education in Russia: Defining Pleasure and Danger for a Fledgling Democratic Society." *Social Science and Medicine* 49: 801–814.

———. 2000. "Health Development Meets the End of State Socialism: Visions of Democratization, Women's Health, and Social Well-Being for Contemporary Russia." *Culture, Medicine, and Psychiatry* 24: 77–100.

———. 2003. "Anthropology, Demography, and the Search for a Critical Analysis of Fertility: Insights from Russia." *American Anthropologist* 105(2): 289–301.

———. 2004a. "'Change Yourself and the Whole World Will Become Kinder'; Russian Activists for Reproductive Health and the Limits of Claims Making for Women." *Medical Anthropology Quarterly* 18(3): 281–304.

———. 2004b. "Gender and Democracy: Strategies for Engagement and Dialogue on Women's Issues in Russia." In *Post-Soviet Women Encountering Transition: Nation Building, Economic Survival, and Civic Activism,* ed. Kathleen Kuehnast and Carol Nechemias, 288–312. Baltimore and Washington, D.C.: Johns Hopkins University Press and Woodrow Wilson International Center for Scholars Press.

———. In press. "Moral Science and the Management of Sexual Revolution in Russia." In *The Moral Object of Sex: Science, Development, and Sexuality in Global Perspective,* ed. Vincanne Adams and Stacy Pigg. Durham, N.C.: Duke University Press.

Ryan, Michael. 1978. *The Organization of Soviet Medical Care.* Oxford: Blackwell.

Saltman, Richard B. 2002. "Regulating Incentives: The Past and Present Role of the State in Health Care Systems." *Social Science and Medicine* 54: 1677–1684.

Sargent, Carolyn, and Thomas Johnson, eds. 1996. *Handbook of Medical Anthropology: Contemporary Theory and Method.* Westport, Conn.: Greenwood Press.

Schecter, Kate. 1992a. "Professionals in Post-Revolutionary Regimes: A Case Study of Soviet Doctors." Ph.D. dissertation, Columbia University.

———. 1992b. "Soviet Socialized Medicine and the Right to Health Care in a Changing Soviet Union." *Human Rights Quarterly* 14(2): 206–215.

———. 2000. "The Politics of Health Care in Russia: The Feminization of Medicine and Other Obstacles to Professionalism." In *Russia's Torn Safety Nets,* ed. M. Field and J. Twigg, 83–100. New York: St. Martin's Press.

Scheper-Hughes, Nancy. 1990. "Three Propositions for a Critically Applied Medical Anthropology." *Social Science and Medicine* 30(2): 189–197.

Semenov, S. S. 1996. "Ostanovit' vymiranie natsii." *Izvestiia,* 13 September.

Shchepin, O. P., and V. C. Nechaev. 1995, "O gosudarstvennykh mekhanizmakh reformy zdravookhraneniia." *Problemy sotsial'noi gigieny, zdravookhraneniia i istorii meditsiny* 1: 34–38.

Shchepin, O. P., et al. 2000. "Osnovnye napravleniia gosudarstvennogo regulirovaniia razvitiia zdravookhraneniia Rossiiskoi Federatsii na 2000–2010 gg." *Problemy sotsial'noi gigieny, zdravookhraneniia i istorii meditsiny* 3: 3–14.

Sheiman, Igor. 1995. "New Methods of Financing and Managing Health Care in the Russian Federation." *Health Policy* 32: 167–180.

Shkolnikov, Vladimir M., Mark G. Field, and Evgueniy Andreev. 2001. "Russia: Socioeconomic Dimensions of the Gender Gap in Mortality." In *Challenging Inequalities in Health,* ed. T. Evans, M. Whitehead, F. Diderichsen, A. Bhuiya, and M. Wirth. New York: Oxford University Press.

Shumilin, Vadim. 2000. "Russians Are Leaving the Volga: Change in Ethnic Balance Is an Extremely Painful Process." *Nezavisimaia gazeta,* 5 September, pp. 9, 11. Reprinted in *CDPSP* 52(36): 13.

Sinyavsky, Andrei. 1990. *Soviet Civilization: A Cultural History.* New York: Arcade Publishing.

Sobo, Elisa. 1995. *Choosing Unsafe Sex: AIDS-Risk Denial among Disadvantaged Women.* Philadelphia: University of Pennsylvania Press.

Solomon, Susan Gross. 1992. "The Demographic Argument in Soviet Debates over the Legalization of Abortion in the 1920s." *Cahiers du Monde Russe et Sovietique* 33(1): 59–82.

Specter, Michael. 1997. "At a Western Outpost of Russia, AIDS Spreads 'Like a Forest Fire.'" *New York Times,* 4 November, pp. A1, A10.

Sperling, Valerie. 1999. *Organizing Women in Contemporary Russia: Engendering Transition.* Cambridge: Cambridge University Press.

Stephenson, Patricia, and Richard Porter. 1994. "Preventing Maternal Mortality in St. Petersburg: Safe Motherhood in a Healthy City." World Health Organization, Healthy Cities Project, WHO Regional Office for Europe (Copenhagen) and St. Petersburg, Russian Federation.

Stone, Linda. 1986. "Primary Health Care for Whom? Village Perspectives from Nepal." *Social Science and Medicine* 22(3): 293–302.

St. Petersburg Maternity Hospital. *Family Births.* Retrieved from www.rody.spb.ru/roddom/rody_home.html, accessed 17 August 2001, pp. 1–13.

Szemere, Anna. 2000. "'We've Kicked the Habit': (Anti) Politics of Art's Autonomy and Transition in Hungary." In *Altering States: Ethnographies of Transition in Eastern Europe and the Former Soviet Union,* ed. Daphne Berdahl, Matti Bunzl, and Martha Lampland, 158–80. Ann Arbor: University of Michigan Press.

Taylor, Carl, and Richard Jolly. 1988. "The Straw Men of Primary Health Care." *Social Science and Medicine* 26(9): 971–977.

Tichonova, L., et al. 1995. "Epidemics of Syphilis in the Russian Federation: Trends, Origins, and Priorities for Control." *Lancet* 350: 210–213.

Togunov, Igor. 1999. "Aspekt lichnosti i otnoshenii v sisteme obespecheniia kachestva meditsinskoi pomoshchi." Retrieved from www.rusmedserv.com/zdrav, accessed 19 March 2002.

Tolstaya, Tatyana. 1990. "Notes from Underground: Soviet Women—Walking the Tightrope." *New York Review of Books,* 31 May, 3–6.

Toth, Olga. 1993. "No Envy, No Pity." In *Gender Politics and Post-Communism: Reflections from Eastern Europe and the Former Soviet Union,* ed. Nanette Funk and Magda Mueller, eds., 213–223. New York: Routledge.

Tronto, Joan C. 1993. *Moral Boundaries: A Political Argument for an Ethic of Care.* New York, Routledge.

Tsyboulsky, Vadim B. 2001. "Patients' Rights in Russia." *European Journal of Health Law* 8: 257–263.

Tulchinsky, Theodore, and Elena Varavikova. 1996. "Addressing the Epidemiologic Transition in the Former Soviet Union: Strategies for Health System and Public Health Reform in Russia." *American Journal of Public Health* 86(3): 313–320.

Twigg, Judyth. 2000. "Unfulfilled Hopes: The Struggle to Reform Russian Health Care and Its Financing." In *Russia's Torn Safety Nets,* ed. M. Field and J. Twigg, 43–64. New York: St. Martin's Press.

———. 2002. "Health Care Reform in Russia: A Survey of Head Doctors and Insurance Administrators." *Social Science and Medicine* 55(12): 2253–2265.

Verdery, Katherine. 1996. *What Was Socialism, and What Comes Next?* Princeton, N.J.: Princeton University Press.

———. 1998. "Transnationalism, Nationalism, Citizenship, and Property: Eastern Europe since 1989." *American Ethnologist* 25(2): 291–306.

———. 1999. "Fuzzy Property: Rights, Power, and Identity in Transylvania's Decollectivization." In *Uncertain Transition: Ethnographies of Change in the Postsocialist World,* ed. M. Burawoy and K. Verdery. Lanham, Md.: Rowman and Littlefield.

———. 2002. "Whither Postsocialism?" In *Postsocialism: Ideals, Ideologies, Practices,* ed. C. M. Hann. London: Routledge.

Vishnevskii, A. G. 1998a. "Russkii krest." Part 1. *Novye Izvestiia,* 24 February.

———. 1998b. "Russkii krest." Part II. *Novye Izvestiia,* 25 February.

———. 1998c. "Russkii krest." Part III. *Novye Izvestiia,* 26 February.

———. 1998d. *Serb i rubl': Konservativnaia modernizatsiia v SSSR.* Moscow: OGI.

Vishnevskii, A.G., ed.

———. 1999. *Naselenie Rossii 1998.* Moscow: Institut Narodnokhoziaistvennogo prognozirovaniia RAN Tsentr demografii i ekologii cheloveka.

———. 2000. *Naselenie Rossii 1999.* Moscow: Institut Narodnokhoziaistvennogo prognozirovaniia RAN Tsentr demografii i ekologii cheloveka.

Visser, A. Ph., N. Bruyniks, and L. Remennick. 1993. "Family Planning in Russia: Experience and Attitudes of Gynecologists." *Advances in Contraception* 9: 93–104.

Volkov, Vadim. 2000. "The Concept of kul'turnost': Notes on the Stalinist Civilizing Process." In *Stalinism: New Directions,* ed. Sheila Fitzpatrick, 210–230. London: Routledge.

Wagner, Marsden. 1994a. "St. Petersburg Healthy Cities Action Plan: 'Giving Birth to a Health Child.'" Unpublished document. Copenhagen: WHO, Regional Office for Europe.

———. 1994b. *Pursuing the Birth Machine: The Search for Appropriate Birth Technology.* Camperdown, Australia: ACE Graphics.

Walsh, Julia A., and Kenneth S. Warren. 1979. "Selective Primary Health Care: An Interim Strategy for Disease Control in Developing Countries." *New England Journal of Medicine* 301(18): 967–974.

Watson, Peggy. 1993a. "The Rise of Masculinism in Eastern Europe." *New Left Review* 198: 71–82.

———. 1993b. "Eastern Europe's Silent Revolution: Gender." *Sociology* 27(3): 471–487.

———. 1997. "Civil Society and the Politics of Difference in Eastern Europe." In *Transitions, Environments, Translations: Feminisms in International Politics,* ed. J. Scott, C. Kaplan, and D. Keates, 21–29. New York: Routledge.

Weare, Katherine. 1992. "The Contribution of Education to Health Promotion." In *Health Promotion: Disciplines and Diversity,* ed. R. Bunton and G. Macdonald, 68–85. New York: Routledge.

Wedel, Janine. 2001. *Collision and Collusion: The Strange Case of Western Aid to Eastern Europe.* New York: St. Martin's Press.

World Bank. 1996. "World Bank Supports Health Services in Russia." Press release, 4 June. Retrieved from http://www.worldbank.org/infoshop.

———. 2002a. "Transition—The First Ten Years: Analysis and Lessons for Eastern Europe and the Former Soviet Union." Washington, D.C.: World Bank.

———. 2002b. "Russian Federation—Health Reform Implementation Project." Retrieved from http://www.worldbank.org/infoshop.

World Health Organization. 1993. "Reforming Services for Mothers and Babies in Eastern Europe: Report on a WHO Consensus Meeting" (St. Petersburg, 9–11 December 1992). Unpublished document. Copenhagen: WHO, Regional Office for Europe.

World Health Organization, Healthy Cities Project. 1993. "St. Petersburg Support Project." Unpublished document. Copenhagen: WHO, Regional Office for Europe.

Yang, Mayfair Mei-hui. 1994. *Gifts, Favors, and Banquets: The Art of Social Relationships in China.* Ithaca, N.Y.: Cornell University Press.

Yurchak, Alexei. 1997. "The Cynical Reason of Late Socialism: Power, Pretense, and the *Anekdote." Public Culture* 9(2): 161–188.

———. 2003. "Soviet Hegemony of Form: Everything Was Forever, Until It Was No More." *Comparative Studies in Society and History* (REF) 45(3): 480–510.

Zakharov, Sergei V. 1999. "Fertility, Nuptiality, and Family Planning in Russia: Problems and Prospects." In *Population under Duress: The Geodemography of Post-Soviet Russia,* ed. G. J. Demko, G. Ioffe, and Z. Zayonchkovskaya, 41–58. Boulder: Westview Press.

Zakharov, Sergei V., and Elena I. Ivanova. 1996. "Fertility Decline and Recent Changes in Russia: On the Threshold of the Second Demographic Transition." In *Russia's Demographic "Crisis,"* ed. J. DaVanzo, 36–82. Santa Monica, Calif.: RAND.

Zarkovic, G., A. Mielck, J. John, and M. Beckmann. 1994. *Reform of the Health Care Systems in Former Socialist Countries: Problems, Options, Scenarios.* Oberschleissheim, Germany: GSF-Forschungszentrum.

Zel'kovich, P. M. 1996. "Trudnye puti reform." *Problemy sotsial'noi gigieny, zdravookhraneniia i istorii meditsiny* 1: 37–39.

INDEX

NEW ANTHROPOLOGIES OF EUROPE

EDITORS
Daphne Berdahl, Matti Bunzl, and Michael Herzfeld

PUBLICATIONS
Algeria in France: Transpolitics, Race, and Nation
Paul A. Silverstein

Locating Bourdieu
Deborah Reed-Danahay

Women's Health in Post-Soviet Russia
Michele Rivkin-Fish

MICHELE RIVKIN-FISH is Associate Professor of Anthropology at
the University of Kentucky.